P9-ARZ-791

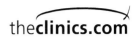

PSYCHIATRIC CLINICS
OF NORTH AMERICA

Recent Research in Personality Disorders

GUEST EDITOR
Joel Paris, MD

September 2008 • Volume 31 • Number 3

SAUNDERS

An Imprint of Elsevier, Inc.
PHILADELPHIA   LONDON   TORONTO   MONTREAL   SYDNEY   TOKYO

W.B. SAUNDERS COMPANY
A Division of Elsevier Inc.

1600 John F. Kennedy Boulevard • Suite 1800 • Philadelphia, PA 19103-2899

http://www.theclinics.com

PSYCHIATRIC CLINICS OF NORTH AMERICA
September 2008
Editor: Sarah E. Barth

Volume 31, Number 3
ISSN 0193-953X
ISBN 13: 978-1-4160-6345-2
ISBN 10: 1-4160-6345-5

Psychiatric Clinics of North America (ISSN 0193-953X) is published quarterly by Elsevier Inc., 360 Park Avenue South, New York, NY 10010-1710. Months of issue are March, June, September, and December. Business and Editorial Offices: 1600 John F. Kennedy Blvd., Suite 1800, Philadelphia, PA 19103-2899. Customer Service Office: 6277 Sea Harbor Drive, Orlando, FL 32887-4800 Periodicals postage paid at New York, NY and additional mailing offices. Subscription prices are $213.00 per year (US individuals), $362.00 per year (US institutions), $107.00 per year (US students/residents), $255.00 per year (Canadian individuals), $440.00 per year (Canadian Institutions), $297.00 per year (foreign individuals), $440.00 per year (foreign institutions), and $149.00 per year (international & Canadian students/residents). Foreign air speed delivery is included in all *Clinics'* subscription prices. All prices are subject to change without notice. **POSTMASTER:** Send address changes to *Psychiatric Clinics of North America*, Elsevier Periodicals Customer Service, 6277 Sea Harbor Drive, Orlando, FL 32887-4800. Customer Service: 1-800-654-2452 (US). From outside of the US, call 1-407-563-6020. Fax: 1-407-363-9661. E-mail: JournalsCustomer Service-usa@elsevier.com.

Reprints. For copies of 100 or more, of articles in this publication, please contact the Commercial Reprints Department, Elsevier Inc., 360 Park Avenue South, New York, New York 10010-1710. Tel.: (212) 633-3813, Fax: (212) 462-1935, E-mail: reprints@elsevier.com.

Psychiatric Clinics of North America is covered in *MEDLINE/PubMed (Index Medicus), Current Contents/Social and Behavioral Sciences, Social Science Citation Index, Embase/Excerpta Medica,* and PsycINFO.

Printed in the United States of America.

Recent Research in Personality Disorders

GUEST EDITOR

JOEL PARIS, MD, Institute of Community and Family Psychiatry, Sir Mortimer B. Davis Jewish General Hospital; and Professor of Psychiatry, McGill University, Montreal, Quebec, Canada

CONTRIBUTORS

IWONA CHELMINSKI, PhD, Clinical Assistant Professor, Department of Psychiatry and Human Behavior, Brown University School of Medicine, Rhode Island Hospital, Bayside Medical Center, Providence, Rhode Island

PATRICIA COHEN, PhD, Professor of Clinical Epidemiology in Psychiatry, Columbia University College of Physicians & Surgeons; and Research Scientist, New York State Psychiatric Institute, New York, New York

ANDREA L. GLENN, MA, Department of Psychology, University of Pennsylvania, Philadelphia, Pennsylvania

MARIANNE GOODMAN, MD, Associate Professor of Psychiatry, The Mount Sinai School of Medicine, New York; and The James J. Peters VA Medical Center, Bronx, New York

MARK F. LENZENWEGER, PhD, Distinguished Professor of Psychology, Department of Psychology, State University of New York at Binghamton, Binghamton; and Adjunct Professor of Psychology in Psychiatry, Department of Psychiatry, Weill Medical College of Cornell University, New York, New York

PAUL S. LINKS, MD, FRCPC, Arthur Sommer Rotenberg Chair in Suicide Studies, Professor of Psychiatry, Department of Psychiatry, University of Toronto, St. Michael's Hospital, Toronto, Ontario, Canada

ELEANOR LIU, PhD, Centre for Addiction and Mental Health, Department of Psychiatry, University of Toronto, Toronto, Ontario, Canada

W. JOHN LIVESLEY, MD, PhD, Professor Emeritus, Department of Psychiatry, University of British Columbia, Vancouver, British Columbia, Canada

JENNIFER RUTH LOWE, MS, Graduate Student, Department of Psychology, University of Kentucky, Lexington, Kentucky

ANTONIA S. NEW, MD, Associate Professor of Psychiatry, The Mount Sinai School of Medicine, New York; and The James J. Peters VA Medical Center, Bronx, New York

JOEL PARIS, MD, Institute of Community and Family Psychiatry, Sir Mortimer B. Davis Jewish General Hospital; and Professor of Psychiatry, McGill University, Montreal, Quebec, Canada

ADRIAN RAINE, PhD, Richard Perry University Professor, Departments of Criminology, Psychiatry, and Psychology, University of Pennsylvania, Philadelphia, Pennsylvania

TED REICHBORN-KJENNERUD, MD, Director, Division of Mental Health, Department of Adult Mental Health, Norwegian Institute of Public Health, Nydalen, Oslo; Professor, Institute of Psychiatry, University of Oslo, Norway; and Adjunct Assistant Professor, Department of Epidemiology, Columbia University, New York, New York

LARRY J. SIEVER, MD, Professor of Psychiatry, The Mount Sinai School of Medicine, New York; and The James J. Peters VA Medical Center, Bronx, New York

ANDREW E. SKODOL, MD, President, Institute for Mental Health Research; and Research Professor of Psychiatry, University of Arizona College of Medicine, Phoenix, Arizona

JOSEPH TRIEBWASSER, MD, Instructor, Department of Psychiatry, The Mount Sinai School of Medicine, New York; and The James J. Peters VA Medical Center, Bronx, New York

JEROME C. WAKEFIELD, PhD, DSW, Professor of Social Work, Professor of Psychiatry, New York University, New York, New York

THOMAS A. WIDIGER, PhD, T. Marshall Hahn Professor of Psychology, Department of Psychology, University of Kentucky, Lexington, Kentucky

DIANE YOUNG, PhD, Clinical Assistant Professor, Department of Psychiatry and Human Behavior, Brown University School of Medicine, Rhode Island Hospital, Bayside Medical Center, Providence, Rhode Island

JUVERIA ZAHEER, MD, Psychiatry Resident, Department of Psychiatry, University of Toronto, Mount Sinai Hospital, Toronto, Ontario, Canada

MARY C. ZANARINI, EdD, Professor of Psychology, Harvard Medical School; and Director, Laboratory for the Study of Adult Development, McLean Hospital, Belmont, Massachusetts

MARK ZIMMERMAN, MD, Associate Professor, Department of Psychiatry and Human Behavior, Brown University School of Medicine, Rhode Island Hospital, Bayside Medical Center, Providence, Rhode Island

Recent Research in Personality Disorders

A proposal made for DSM-IV was to include a means with which to provide a dimensional profile of a patient in terms of the diagnostic categories. However, a suggestion of the DSM-V Research Planning Conference on personality disorders was to develop a more fundamental revision through an integration of alternative dimensional models of personality disorder and general personality structure. A purpose of the current article is to provide this proposal. Also discussed is a primary concern with respect to the implementation of any such dimensional model: clinical utility. Discussed in particular are concerns regarding feasibility and treatment implications.

The harmful dysfunction analysis of mental disorder is used to assess whether traits are indicative of personality disorder, and the ways such an inference can go wrong. Personality is an overall organization that allows the organism to accomplish basic goals within the constraints of its basic traits and specific intentional states. Extreme traits can be negative or "dysfunctional" in the sense that they interfere with the achievement of socially or personally valued goals; however, they are not necessarily dysfunctions or disorders in the biological or medical sense. Thus, no sheer assessment of a set of traits can offer sufficient information for a diagnosis of personality disorder. Nor do criteria such as maladaptiveness, impairment, or clinical significance necessarily transform a trait into a personality disorder. The DSM's most plausible suggestion for judging when traits are dysfunctions, inflexibility, is also problematic because many nondisordered traits are inflexible as well.

The prevalence of personality disorders (PDs) in the nonclinical community population was largely unknown through the early 1990s. Over the past 10 years the epidemiology of PD in the community has been resolved through the study of large, nonclinical populations that have used validated structured psychiatric interviews designed specifically for PDs. The median prevalence for "any PD" is 10.6%, which is reasonably consistent across six major studies spanning three nations. Because 1 in 10 people suffers from a diagnosable PD and the disorders are associated with high levels of service use, it follows that personality pathology represents a major public health concern, a major research target for psychopathologists, and a consuming focus for clinicians.

Community-based epidemiological studies of psychiatric disorders provide important information about the public health burden of these problems; however, because seeking treatment is related to a number of clinical and demographic factors, studies of the frequency and correlates of psychiatric disorders in the general population should be replicated in clinical populations to provide the practicing clinician with information that might have more direct clinical utility. Diagnosing co-occuring personality disorders in psychiatric patients with an Axis I disorder is clinically important because of their association with the duration, recurrence, and outcome of Axis I disorders. This article reviews clinical epidemiological studies of personality disorders and finds that in studies using semi-structured diagnostic interviews, approximately half of the patients interviewed have a personality disorder. Thus, as a group, personality disorders are among the most frequent disorders treated by psychiatrists.

This review of the literature on genetic contributions to the etiology of personality disorders broadly follows the DSM classification, and begins by evaluating the current evidence for genetic influences on the DSM axis II disorders. One of the most exciting directions in psychiatric genetics is the rapidly developing field of molecular genetic studies aiming to identify specific genes correlated with psychiatric phenotypes. Personality disorders, like most other psychiatric diagnostic categories, are etiologically complex, which implies that they are influenced by several genes and several environmental factors. The interplay between genes and the environment is a field that is receiving increasing attention and is addressed both in relation to quantitative and molecular methods.

> While it is premature to provide a simple model for the vulnerability to the development of either borderline (BPD) or schizotypal (SPD) personality disorder, it is clear that these heritable disorders lend themselves to fruitful neurobiological exploration. The most promising findings in BPD suggest that a diminished top-down control of affective responses, which is likely to relate to deceased responsiveness of specific midline regions of prefrontal cortex, may underlie the affective hyperresponsiveness in this disorder. In addition, genetic and neuroendocrine and molecular neuro-imaging findings point to a role for serotonin in this affective disinhibition. Clearly SPD falls within the schizophrenia spectrum, but precisely the nature of what predicts full-blown schizophrenia as opposed to the milder symptoms of SPD is not yet clear.

> Numerous studies have tackled the complex challenge of understanding the neural substrates of psychopathy, revealing that brain abnormalities exist on several levels and in several structures. As we discover more about complex neural networks, it becomes increasingly difficult to clarify how these systems interact with each other to produce the distinct pattern of behavioral and personality characteristics observed in psychopathy. The authors review the recent research on the neurobiology of psychopathy, beginning with molecular neuroscience work and progressing to the level of brain structures and their connectivity. Potential factors that may affect the development of brain impairments, as well as how some systems may be targeted for potential treatment, are discussed.

> The evidence is surprisingly strong that even early adolescent personality disorders or elevated personality disorder symptoms have a broad range of negative effects well into adulthood, for the most part comparable to or even larger than those of Axis I disorders. Current evidence suggests that the most severe long-term prognosis is associated with borderline and schizotypal PDs and elevated symptoms. And of course, childhood conduct disorder is in a peculiar status, disappearing in adulthood to be manifest as a very severe disorder—antisocial PD—in a minority of those with the adolescent disorder.

Part IV - Outcome

The notion of personality disorders (PDs) as stable disorders has persisted despite traditional follow-up studies showing that fewer than 50% of patients diagnosed with PDs retained these diagnoses over time. Because these studies had methodological limitations, four more rigorous large-scale studies of the naturalistic course of PDs have been conducted. The results indicate (1) personality psychopathology improves over time at unexpectedly significant rates; (2) maladaptive personality traits are more stable than PD diagnoses; (3) although personality psychopathology improves, residual effects can be seen in the form of persistent functional impairment, continuing behavioral problems, reduced future quality of life, and ongoing Axis I psychopathology; (4) improvement in personality psychopathology may eventually be associated with reduction in ongoing personal and social burden.

Borderline personality disorder is a slow-moving disorder. Most patients who have borderline personality disorder improve over time; however, the reasons for this change are unclear. Therapy as usual and the reparations that adult life offers can facilitate these changes.

Part V - Treatment

The objective of this review is to examine clinical trials of the treatment of personality disorders (PDs). The method is a narrative review of published controlled trials of psychotherapy and pharmacotherapy. Results show that a variety of methods reduce impulsivity, with less striking results for affective instability. There is good support for well-structured methods of psychotherapy, mainly in borderline personality disorder (BPD), but evidence for the efficacy of pharmacotherapy is weak. Research on other PD categories is sparse.

This article examines the association between suicidal behavior and personality disorders. It updates the review of epidemiological evidence for the association between suicidal behavior and suicide in individuals who have a personality disorder diagnosis, particularly in borderline personality disorder (BPD). The second part of the article presents new empirical evidence that characterizes suicidal behavior in patients who have BPD, specifically examining patient characteristics that differentiate patients who have BPD with a history of high versus low lethality suicide attempts. Finally, the article discusses the approach to a patient who has BPD and presents to the emergency department because of an increased risk of suicide.

Part VI - Future Directions

An examination of current research trends needs to consider both the prerequisites for research and the specific research directions needed to arrive at a more systematic understanding of the etiology, development, course, and treatment of personality disorder. Important prerequisites are improved phenotypes and more sophisticated research designs to explicate mechanisms specific to the various patterns of personality disorder. Specific research themes with promise are systematic studies of gene-environment interplay, investigations of biological substrates, and longitudinal studies capable of generating information on how the different domains of personality pathology change over time. There also needs to be a new generation of treatment research that is less concerned with comparing the outcome of treatments that often seem modest in effects and limited in scope and more concerned with identifying the most effective treatment methods for each domain of psychopathology. Along with these developments it is also important that research pays more attention to how the integrative processes within personality become dysfunctional in personality disorder.

FORTHCOMING ISSUES

RECENT ISSUES

Preface

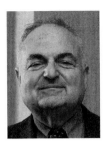

Joel Paris, MD
Guest Editor

Research in personality disorders is moving forward rapidly. This issue of the *Psychiatric Clinics of North America* summarizes the advancing edge of our knowledge.

The first question concerns how to diagnose personality disorders. Much ink has been spent on this subject. On the one hand, disorders may be pathologic exaggerations of normal personality traits. For this reason some have suggested that the current Axis II categories be replaced with dimensional scores (see article by Widiger and Lowe). We need to establish a clearer boundary between normal and abnormal personality patterns (see article by Wakefield). On the other hand, several of the existing categories show symptoms not seen in normal people, such as the chronic suicidality of patients who have borderline personality. Moreover, most of the research described in this issue is based on categories. It remains important that both antisocial personality (or psychopathy) and borderline personality have large and important research traditions of their own.

A second research question concerns the prevalence of personality disorders. Recent years have seen a large number of epidemiologic studies, all of which suggest that personality disorders are very common in community populations (see article by Lenzenweger). Personality disorders are even more common in clinical populations, even if they often go unrecognized (see article by Zimmerman, Chelminski, and Young).

A third question concerns the etiology of personality disorders. Although much remains unknown, researchers are chipping away at these problems. Approaches include genetic studies (see article by Reichborn-Kjennrud), imaging studies (see articles by New, Goodman, Triebwasser, and Siever and by Glenn and Raine). Another important research method involves longitudinal

0193-953X/08/$ – see front matter
doi:10.1016/j.psc.2008.03.002

follow-ups of children to determine the precursors and predictors of personality disorders (see article by Cohen).

A fourth question concerns the outcome of personality disorders. Whereas in the past these conditions were seen as lifelong and chronic, research has drawn a much more hopeful picture (see articles by Skodol and Zanarini).

A fifth question concerns treatment. Although clinical trials of therapy for personality disorders are encouraging, patients do not respond to methods of treatment that work for other patients (see article by Paris). Perhaps the most challenging issue for clinicians in treating personality disorders is suicidality; but we are getting a better understanding of how to manage these problems (see article by Zaheer, Links, and Liu).

The snapshot presented in this issue should not obscure the need for further research to illuminate many unresolved issues (see article by Livesley). When we learn how to understand and treat personality disorders better, these patients may no longer be seen as unmanageable and will no longer be given other diagnoses.

Joel Paris, MD
Institute of Community and Family Psychiatry
Sir Mortimer B. Davis Jewish General Hospital
Department of Psychiatry, McGill University
4333 Cote Ste. Catherine
Montreal, Quebec H3T 1E4, Canada

E-mail address: joel.paris@mcgill.ca

A Dimensional Model of Personality Disorder: Proposal for DSM-V

Thomas A. Widiger, PhD*, Jennifer Ruth Lowe, MS

Department of Psychology, University of Kentucky, 106-B Kastle Hall,
Lexington, KY 40506-0044, USA

The question of whether personality disorders are discrete clinical conditions or arbitrary distinctions along dimensions of general personality functioning has been a longstanding issue. Proposals for a dimensional model have been made throughout the history of the American Psychiatric Association's (APA) diagnostic manual [1]. In 1999, a DSM-V Research Planning Conference was held under joint sponsorship of the APA and the National Institute of Mental Health (NIMH), the purpose of which was to set research priorities that might affect future classifications. The impetus for this conference was the frustration with the existing nomenclature.

> "In the more than 30 years since the introduction of the Feighner criteria by Robins and Guze, which eventually led to DSM-III, the goal of validating these syndromes and discovering common etiologies has remained elusive. Despite many proposed candidates, not one laboratory marker has been found to be specific in identifying any of the DSM-defined syndromes. Epidemiologic and clinical studies have shown extremely high rates of comorbidities among the disorders, undermining the hypothesis that the syndromes represent distinct etiologies. Furthermore, epidemiologic studies have shown a high degree of short-term diagnostic instability for many disorders. With regard to treatment, lack of treatment specificity is the rule rather than the exception [2]".

DSM-V Research Planning Work Groups were formed to develop white papers to impact the development of the diagnostic manual. The Nomenclature Work Group concluded that it is "important that consideration be given to advantages and disadvantages of basing part or all of DSM-V on dimensions rather than categories" [3]. They recommended in particular that initial efforts toward a dimensional model of classification be developed for the personality disorders. "If a dimensional system of personality performs well and is acceptable to clinicians, it might then be appropriate to explore dimensional approaches in other domains" [3]. The white paper concerning

*Corresponding author. E-mail address: widiger@uky.edu (T.A. Widiger).

0193-953X/08/$ – see front matter
doi:10.1016/j.psc.2008.03.008

personality disorders provided the rationale and empirical support for converting this section of the manual to a dimensional classification [4]. The white papers were followed by a series of DSM-V Research Planning Conferences (see www.DSM5.org; for a summary of each conference). It was the decision of the executive committee governing these conferences to have the first devoted to setting a research agenda that would be most useful and effective in leading the field toward a dimensional classification of personality disorder [5].

One proposal for DSM-V is simply to provide a dimensional profile of the existing (or somewhat revised) diagnostic categories [6]. A personality disorder would be characterized as prototypic if all of the diagnostic criteria are met, moderately present if one or two criteria beyond the threshold are present, threshold if the patient just barely meets the diagnostic threshold, subthreshold if symptoms are present but are just below diagnostic threshold, traits if no more than one to three symptoms are present, and absent if no diagnostic criteria are present. This proposal was in fact made for DSM-IV [7] but at the time it was considered to be too radical of a shift [8]. It is now perhaps the more conservative of the proposals for DSM-V [9].

A dimensional classification of the existing diagnostic constructs would be beneficial in shifting clinicians somewhat toward a more dimensional manner of conceptualization. It would encourage practitioners to provide a more comprehensive and precise description of a patient's profile of maladaptive personality functioning and would discourage fruitless differential diagnoses of overlapping constructs [6,7].

However, a limitation of this proposed revision is that clinicians would continue to be describing patients in terms of markedly heterogeneous and overlapping constructs. A profile description of a patient in terms the antisocial, borderline, dependent, histrionic, and other DSM-IV-TR (or DSM-V) constructs would essentially reify the excessive diagnostic co-occurrence that is currently being obtained [10–12]. In other words, the problem of excessive diagnostic co-occurrence would not in fact be solved. It would simply be accepted as an inherent limitation of the diagnostic system. This is comparable to the decision made by the authors of DSM-III-R [13] to address the problematic heterogeneity of the diagnostic categories by abandoning monothetic criterion sets that required homogeneity and converting to polythetic criterion sets that accepted the existence of the problematic heterogeneity [14].

A suggestion of the DSM-V Research Planning Conference on personality disorders was to develop a more fundamental revision to the nomenclature through an integration of alternative dimensional models of personality disorder and general personality structure [15]. A format for such a hierarchical model was provided, but no specific, concrete proposal was presented. The purpose of the current paper is in part to provide this proposal. We also discuss what is perhaps the primary concern with respect to the implementation of any such dimensional model: clinical utility.

FIVE-FACTOR MODEL OF PERSONALITY DISORDER

A fundamental revision of the existing nomenclature would be to integrate the psychiatric classification of personality disorder with the predominant dimensional model of general personality structure, the five-factor model (FFM) [9]. The FFM consists of five broad domains of general personality functioning: neuroticism versus emotional stability, extraversion versus introversion, openness versus closedness to experience, agreeableness versus antagonism, and conscientiousness versus irresponsibility. The FFM was derived originally through studies of the trait terms within the English language. This lexical paradigm was guided by the compelling hypothesis that what is of most importance, interest, or meaning to persons for describing themselves and others is encoded within the language. Language can be understood as a sedimentary deposit of the observations of persons over the thousands of years of the language's development and transformation. The most important domains of personality functioning are those with the most number of trait terms to describe and differentiate the various manifestations and nuances of that domain, and the structure of personality is evident by the empirical relationships among the trait terms. The initial lexical studies were conducted with the English language, and these investigations converged well onto a five-factor structure [16]. Subsequent lexical studies have been conducted in many additional languages (eg, German, Dutch, Czech, Polish, Russian, Italian, Spanish, Hebrew, Hungarian, Turkish, Korean, and Filipino) and these have confirmed reasonably well the existence of the five broad domains [17]. The five broad domains have been differentiated into more specific facets by Costa and McCrae [18] on the basis of their development of and research with the NEO Personality Inventory-Revised (NEO PI-R), by far the most commonly used and heavily researched measure of the FFM.

An advantage of this integrative model is the development of a uniform classification of personality and personality disorder that would cover both normal and abnormal personality functioning within a single, common structure, as well as bringing to our understanding of personality disorders a considerable amount of basic science research supporting behavior genetics [19], molecular genetics [20,21], childhood antecedents [22,23], temporal stability across the life span [24], and universality [17,25]. This is a scientific foundation that is sorely lacking for the existing nomenclature [9]. As acknowledged by even proponents of the existing personality disorder diagnostic constructs, "similar construct validity has been more elusive to attain with the current DSM-IV personality disorder categories" [26].

A significant limitation of an FFM of personality disorder, however, is the absence of obvious face validity for clinical application, at least as the FFM is currently described within the NEO PI-R. For example, some of the scale titles of the NEO PI-R lack a strong or at times even apparent relevance to personality disorder. This is because the initial studies were conducted within nonclinical samples and the scales were therefore written with respect to the more normal, common range of expression of each dimension rather than with regard to the extreme or maladaptive expressions [18]. For example, NEO PI-R positive emotionality does not itself have strong face validity for clinical application, yet maladaptively low positive emotionality is the anhedonia that is central to the schizoid personality disorder and maladaptively high positive emotionality concerns the excessive euphoria, gaiety, and dyscontrolled, hypomania evident in some cases of the histrionic personality disorder [27]. Similarly, NEO PI-R compliance does not adequately convey the maladatively extreme variant of meek submissiveness (evident in many persons with a dependent personality disorder), nor at the opposite pole the oppositionalism (evident in passive-aggressive persons) or aggressiveness (evident in antisocial persons).

Table 1 provides an abbreviated, tabular summary of adaptive and maladaptive variants of all 60 poles of all 30 facets of the FFM, adapted from a modification of a brief rating form for the assessment of the FFM, the Five-Factor Model Rating Form [28]. An inspection of the maladaptive poles of each of the 30 facets will indicate the breadth of maladaptive personality functioning covered by the FFM. Studies within clinical and non-clinical samples have now documented that all of the DSM-IV-TR personality disorder symptomatology can be understood as maladaptive variants of the domains and facets of the FFM [29–32]. As acknowledged by Livesley [33], "multiple studies provide convincing evidence that the DSM personality disorders diagnoses show a systematic relationship to the five factors and that all categorical diagnoses of DSM can be accommodated within the five-factor framework." As expressed by Clark [10], "the five-factor model of personality is widely accepted as representing the higher-order structure of both normal and abnormal personality traits." These are compelling endorsements, as they are provided by authors of alternative dimensional models [34,35].

Table 2 provides a description of the DSM-IV-TR personality disorders in terms of the FFM, adapted from surveys of both clinicians [36] and researchers [37]. It is evident from Table 2 that each personality disorder can be described in terms of the facets of the FFM. The FFM descriptions in fact go beyond the DSM-IV-TR criterion sets to provide fuller, more comprehensive descriptions of each personality disorder. For example, the FFM includes the traits of DSM-IV-TR antisocial personality disorder (deception, exploitation, aggression, irresponsibility, negligence, rashness, angry hostility, impulsivity, excitement-seeking, and assertiveness; see Tables 1 and 2), and goes beyond DSM-IV-TR to include additional traits within the widely popular Psychopathy Checklist-Revised (PCL-R; Ref. [38]), such as glib charm (low self-consciousness), arrogance, and lack of empathy (tough-minded callousness) and goes even further to include traits of psychopathy emphasized originally by Cleckley [39] but not included within either the DSM-IV-TR or the PCL-R, such as low anxiousness and low vulnerability or fearlessness. The FFM has the social withdrawal evident in the avoidant, schizoid, and schizotypal personality disorders, but also the anxiousness and self-consciousness of the avoidant, the anhedonia that is considered to be specific to the schizoid, and the cognitive-perceptual aberrations of the schizotypal. The FFM has the intense attachment needs, the deference, and the self-conscious anxiousness of the dependent, the perfectionism and workaholism of the obsessive-compulsive, and the fragile vulnerability and emotional dysregulation of the borderline. The FFM also goes beyond the DSM-IV-TR nomenclature to include closed-mindedness (evident in racist, prejudicial persons; Ref. [40]) and alexithymia [41].

CLINICAL UTILITY

One of the fundamental concerns regarding a shift to a dimensional classification of personality disorder is clinical utility. This concern is perhaps somewhat ironic as it is not particularly clear that the existing diagnostic categories have compelling clinical utility. Verheul [42] systematically reviewed various components of clinical utility for both the categorical and dimensional models and concluded, "overall, the categorical system has the least evidence for clinical utility, especially with respect to coverage, reliability, subtlety, and clinical decision-making." In an international survey of psychiatrists and psychologists, Maser and colleagues [43] indicated that the section of the diagnostic manual with which respondents were most dissatisfied was the personality disorders. Maser and colleagues did not determine precisely the nature of the clinicians' dissatisfaction, but the heterogeneity of diagnostic membership, the lack of precision in description, the excessive diagnostic co-occurrence, the failure to lead to a specific diagnosis, the reliance on the "not otherwise specified" wastebasket diagnosis, and the unstable and arbitrary diagnostic boundaries, are likely to be sources of considerable frustration for the clinician [9].

Nevertheless, as First [44] argued in his rejoinder to proposals for converting the psychiatric diagnostic categories into dimensions, "the most important obstacle standing in the way of its implementation in DSM-V (and beyond) is questions about clinical utility." Two concerns that have been raised in particular are feasibility and treatment implications.

Feasibility

Clinicians may understandably respond with a deep breath of concern upon first inspection of Table 1. Many clinicians would find it daunting to conceive of becoming familiar with both the adaptive and maladaptive variants of all 60 poles of all 30 facets of the FFM. In addition, a few of the facets or specific poles lack substantially compelling clinical relevance even at the maladaptive level. For instance, maladaptively high and low openness to aesthetics are unlikely, to say the least, to be a significant focus of treatment in most clinical settings. A classification system that is considered to be so extensive and at times irrelevant is unlikely to be used effectively, reliably, or validly [44].

Fig. 1 provides a simpler version. The dimensional classification of personality disorder provided in Fig. 1 is a simplification of the FFM proposal in a number of ways. First, the adaptive behaviors are confined to just the five broad domains rather than the 30 facets. In addition, the maladaptive facets have been reduced from 60 to just 26. This reduction was achieved in part

Table 1

Adaptive and maladaptive variants of the five-factor model as presented in five-factor form

	Maladaptively high	Normal high	Normal low	Maladaptively low
NEUROTICISM				
Anxiousness	Fearful, anxious	Vigilant, worrisome, jittery, wary	Relaxed, calm	Oblivious to signs of threat
Angry hostility	Rageful	Brooding, resentful, defiant	Even-tempered	Won't even protest exploitation
Depressiveness	Depressed, suicidal	Pessimistic, discouraged	Not easily discouraged	Unrealistic, overly optimistic
Self-consciousness	Uncertain of self or identity	Self-conscious, embarrassed	Self-assured, charming	Glib, shameless
Impulsivity	Unable to resist impulses	Self-indulgent	Restrained	Overly restrained
Vulnerability	Helpless, emotionally unstable	Vulnerable, fragile	Resilient	Fearless, feels invincible
EXTRAVERSION				
Warmth	Intense attachments	Affectionate, warm	Formal, reserved	Cold, distant
Gregariousness	Attention-seeking	Sociable, outgoing, personable	Independent	Isolated
Assertiveness	Dominant, pushy	Assertive, forceful	Passive	Submissive
Activity	Frantic	Energetic	Slow-paced	Lethargic, sedentary
Excitement-Seeking	Reckless, foolhardy	Adventurous	Cautious	Dull, listless
Positive emotions	Melodramatic, manic	High-spirited, cheerful, joyful	Placid, sober, serious	Grim, anhedonic
OPENNESS				
Fantasy	Unrealistic, lives in fantasy	Imaginative	Practical, realistic	Concrete
Aesthetics	Bizarre interests	Aesthetic interests	Minimal aesthetic interests	Disinterested
Feelings	Intense, in turmoil	Self-aware, expressive	Constricted, blunted	Alexithymic

Facet				
Actions	Eccentric	Unconventional	Predictable	Mechanized, stuck in routine
Ideas	Peculiar, weird	Creative, curious	Pragmatic	Closed-minded
Values	Radical	Open, flexible	Traditional	Dogmatic, moralistically intolerant
AGREEABLENESS				
Trust	Gullible	Trusting	Cautious, skeptical	Cynical, suspicious
Straightforwardness	Guileless	Honest, forthright	Savvy, cunning, shrewd	Deceptive, dishonest, manipulative
Altruism	Self-sacrificial, selfless	Giving, generous	Frugal, withholding	Greedy, exploitative
Compliance	Yielding, docile, meek	Cooperative, obedient, deferential	Critical, contrary	Combative, aggressive
Modesty	Self-effacing, self-denigrating	Humble, modest, unassuming	Confident, self-assured	Boastful, pretentious, arrogant
Tender-mindedness	Overly soft-hearted	Empathic, sympathetic, gentle	Strong, tough	Callous, merciless, ruthless
CONSCIENTIOUSNESS				
Competence	Perfectionistic	Efficient, resourceful	Casual	Disinclined, lax
Order	Preoccupied with organization	Organized, methodical	Disorganized	Careless, sloppy, haphazard
Dutifulness	Rigidly principled	Dependable, reliable, responsible	Easy-going, capricious	Irresponsible, undependable, immoral
Achievement	Workaholic	Purposeful, diligent, ambitious	Carefree, content	Aimless, shiftless, desultory
Self-discipline	Single-minded doggedness	Self-disciplined, willpower	Leisurely	Negligent, hedonistic
Deliberation	Ruminative, indecisive	Thoughtful, reflective, circumspect	Quick to make decisions	Hasty, rash

Table 2
DSM-IV-TR personality disorders from the perspective of the five-factor model of general personality structure

	PRN	SZD	SZT	ATS	BDL	HST	NCS	AVD	DPD	OCP
NEUROTICISM (VERSUS EMOTIONAL STABILITY)										
Anxiousness (versus unconcerned)			H	L	H			H	H	H
Angry hostility (versus dispassionate)	H			H	H		H			
Depressiveness (versus optimistic)					H					
Self-Consciousness (versus shameless)			H	L	H	L	L	H	H	
Impulsivity (versus restrained)				H	H	H				L
Vulnerability (versus fearless)				L	H			H	H	
EXTRAVERSION (VERSUS INTROVERSION)										
Warmth (versus coldness)	L	L	L				L		H	
Gregariousness (versus withdrawal)	L	L	L	H		H		L		
Assertiveness (versus submissiveness)				H			H	L	L	
Activity (versus passivity)		L		H		H				
Excitement-seeking (versus dullness)		L		H		H	H	L		L
Positive emotionality (versus anhedonia)	L	L				H				
OPENNESS (VERSUS CLOSEDNESS)										
Fantasy (versus concrete)						H				
Aesthetics (versus disinterest)										
Feelings (versus alexithymia)		L			H	H	L			L
Actions (versus routine)	L	L		H	H	H	H	L		L
Ideas (versus closed-minded)			H							L
Values (versus dogmatic)	L									L
AGREEABLENESS (VERSUS ANTAGONISM)										
Trust (versus mistrust)	L		L	L	L	H	L		H	
Straightforwardness (versus deception)	L		L				L			

(continued on next page)

Table 2
(continued)

	PRN	SZD	SZT	ATS	BDL	HST	NCS	AVD	DPD	OCP
Altruism (versus exploitation)				L			L			
Compliance (versus opposition, aggression)	L			L	L		L		H	
Modesty (versus arrogance)				L			L	H	H	
Tender-mindedness (versus tough-minded)	L			L			L			
CONSCIENTIOUSNESS (VERSUS DISINHIBITION)										
Competence (versus ineptitude)					L				L	H
Order (versus disordered)			L							H
Dutifulness (versus irresponsibility)				L						H
Achievement-striving (versus lackadaisical)										H
Self-discipline (versus negligence)				L		L				H
Deliberation (versus rashness)				L	L	L				H

Abbreviations: ATS, antisocial; AVD, avoidant; BDL, borderline; DPD, dependent; H, high; HST, histrionic; L, low; NCS, narcissistic; OCP, obsessive-compulsive; PRN, paranoid; SZD, schizoid; and SZT, schizotypal.

by eliminating poles of facets that were considered to be too infrequent or obscure for most clinical use (eg, maladaptively high straightforwardness and openness to aesthetics). Emphasis for inclusion was placed on facets from alternative dimensional models that would have particular clinical relevance, consistent with the DSM-V Research Planning Conference recommendation to work toward a common, integrative model [15].

This proposed dimensional model for DSM-V begins with the description of the person in terms of general personality functioning at the level of the five broad domains of the FFM (eg, conscientiousness). Each of these five broad domains would be assessed with five to seven diagnostic criteria comparable to the format currently used within DSM-IV but this time referring to normal, adaptive behavior. The classification thereby provides information concerning a patient's personality strengths (as well as the deficits assessed at the facet level).

The inclusion of normal, adaptive personality traits is useful in a number of regards. First, it can be helpful in reducing the stigma of a mental disorder diagnosis [45]. Persons are not just provided a diagnostic category characterizing their personality disorder, as if they have no personality traits or strengths beyond the disorder. Personality disorders are relatively unique in concerning ego-syntonic aspects of the self, or one's characteristic manner of thinking, feeling, behaving and relating to others pretty much every day throughout one's

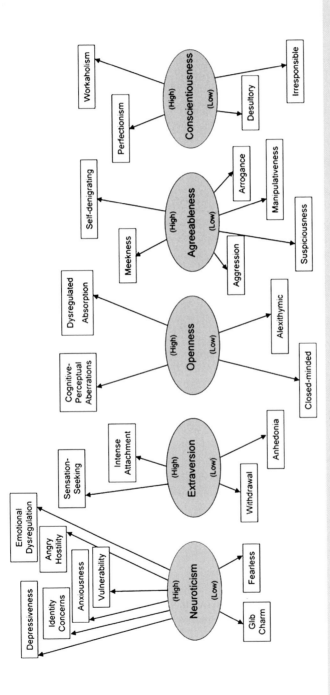

Fig. 1. Dimensional model of personality disorder proposal for DSM-V.

adult life [46]. In this regard, a personality disorder diagnosis can be quite stig-matizing, suggesting that who you are and always have been is itself a mental disorder. The proposal for DSM-V presented in Fig. 1 provides a more com-plete description of each person's unique self that recognizes and appreciates that the person is more than just the personality disorder and that there are aspects to the self that can be adaptive, even commendable, despite the presence of the personality disorder. Some of these strengths may also be quite relevant to treatment, such as openness to experience indicating an interest in exploratory psychotherapy, an agreeableness and extraversion that suggest an engagement in group therapy, or a conscientiousness that indicates a willingness and ability to adhere to the demands and rigor of dialectical behavior therapy [47].

The abbreviated version does naturally fail to include all of the maladaptive traits present within the FFM, as presented in Table 1. With any simplification some amount of information will be lost. Nevertheless, clinicians can readily access the additional information through various measures of the FFM that provide a more comprehensive assessment of all of the FFM facets [32].

The presence of 26 facets might still seem daunting, but it is important to appreciate that each of these clinical constructs are substantially easier to assess than the DSM-IV-TR personality disorders as the latter involve complex com-binations and constellations of these constructs [9,34,35]. In addition, the mal-adaptive facets are only assessed if there is an elevation on a respective domain. For instance, if the person is elevated in agreeableness, one would only assess for the maladaptive meekness and self-denigration. One would not need to assess for the suspiciousness, manipulation, aggression, or arrogance of malad-aptively low agreeableness. In addition, if the person was neither significantly high nor low in agreeableness, one would not have to consider any one of the six maladaptive variants of agreeableness or antagonism. An FFM assessment of personality disorder generally takes half the amount of time as an assessment of the DSM-IV-TR personality disorders, as much of the administration of a personality disorder semi-structured interview is spent in the assessment of diagnostic criteria that are not present [32]. This waste of time is diminished substantially by the FFM approach through the screening process of assessing whether the person is high or low in the five broad domains of general person-ality functioning.

Treatment Implications

An additional utility concern is the implications for treatment [42]. The FFM, at least as it is presented in the NEO PI-R, can appear to be limited in its impli-cations for treatment. However, the factor analytic development of the FFM does in fact provide a more conceptually (as well as empirically) coherent struc-ture. Extraversion and agreeableness are the domains of interpersonal related-ness, neuroticism is the domain of emotional instability and dysregulation, conscientiousness is the domain of work-related behavior and responsibility, and openness is the domain of cognitive intellect, curiosity, and creativity [18,29]. Personality disorders are diagnosed when the maladaptive personality traits result in "clinically significant distress or impairment in social, occupational, or other important areas of functioning" [48]. The FFM structure is nicely organized with respect to these relatively specific areas of dysfunction.

The FFM extraversion and agreeableness domains concern the social, interpersonal dysfunction, an area of functioning that is particularly relevant to relationship quality both outside and within the therapy office. Interpersonal models of therapy, marital-family therapy, and group therapy would be confined largely to these two domains, or at least they would have the most specific and explicit implications for these forms of treatment. In contrast, neuroticism provides information with respect to the "distress" of personality disorder, or more precisely the depression, anxiousness, anger, and emotional dyscontrol, often targets for pharmacologic interventions (as well as other modalities of treatment). There are very clear pharmacologic implications for mood and anxiety dysregulation but little to none for maladaptive antagonism or introversion, the interpersonal domains of the FFM. Maladaptively high openness implies cognitive-perceptual aberrations and dysregulated absorption (eg, dissociation), which have pharmacologic implications that are quite different from those of neuroticism. The domain of conscientiousness is, in contrast to agreeableness and extraversion, the domain of most specific relevance to occupational dysfunction, or impairments concerning work, employment, and career. Maladaptively high levels involve workaholism, perfectionism, and compulsivity; low levels involve laxness, negligence, and irresponsibility. There are even specific pharmacologic treatment implications for low conscientiousness (eg, comparable to those used for attention-deficits and hyperactivity), although, as yet, none for maladaptively high conscientiousness (and for which there may never be). In sum, the structure of the FFM is commensurate with much more specific treatment implications than the existing diagnostic categories.

As expressed by the chair of DSM-V, for the existing diagnostic categories, "lack of treatment specificity is the rule rather than the exception" [2]. It is telling that it has been over 10 years since the American Psychiatric Association began publishing practice guidelines for the diagnostic categories of DSM-IV-TR and, as yet, treatment guidelines have been developed for only 1 of the 10 personality disorder diagnostic categories [49]. The reason is straightforward: there have been no adequate empirical studies on the treatment of the avoidant, schizoid, paranoid, histrionic, narcissistic, obsessive-compulsive, or dependent personality disorders. There is very little that can be said empirically regarding their treatment.

It is not that the DSM-IV-TR personality disorders are untreatable. There are a number of excellent texts to help clinicians treat personality disorders [50–56] and "psychotherapy studies indicate that, as a group, personality disorders improve with treatment" [57]. There is compelling empirical support to indicate that a meaningful response to treatment does occur [57,58].

However, what is also evident from this research is that treatment does not address or focus on the entire personality structure [54,55]. Clinicians treat, for instance, the affective instability or the self-mutilation of persons diagnosed with borderline personality disorder. Effective change occurs with respect to these components rather than the entire, global construct. One of the empirically supported treatments for borderline personality disorder is dialectical behavior therapy (DBT) [49]. Research has demonstrated that DBT is an effective treatment for many of the components of this personality disorder, but it is evident to even the proponents of this clinical approach that the treatment is not entirely comprehensive in its effectiveness [59]. DBT has been particularly effective with respect to decreasing self-harm and angry hostility, but not with other aspects of borderline psychopathology, such as hopelessness [60]. These different components of borderline personality disorder are readily identified and distinguished in the FFM of personality disorder (see Table 1). It is difficult to imagine clinicians not finding useful a classification system that concerns explicitly their focus of treatment, such as cognitive-perceptual aberrations, anxiousness, emotional dysregulation, intense attachment, meekness, and workaholism (see Fig. 1).

SUMMARY

Work is now beginning on DSM-V. It is hoped that the Personality Disorders Work Group and the DSM-V Task Force will appreciate the validity and utility of at least including a model comparable to the one proposed herein. An FFM dimensional model of personality disorder would describe abnormal functioning with the same model and language used to describe general personality structure. It would transfer to the psychiatric nomenclature a wealth of knowledge concerning the origins, development, and stability of the dispositions that underlie personality disorder; it would bring with it well-validated and researched instruments and methods of assessment; it would facilitate the development of a more truly universal diagnostic system; and it would represent a significant step toward a rapprochement and integration of psychiatry with psychology.

References

[1] Widiger TA, Simonsen E. The American Psychiatric Association's research agenda for the DSM-V. J Personal Disord 2005;19:103–9.

[2] Kupfer DJ, First MB, Regier DE. Introduction. In: Kupfer DJ, First MB, Regier DE, editors. A research agenda for DSM-V. Washington, DC: American Psychiatric Association; 2002. p. xv–xxiii.

[3] Rounsaville BJ, Alarcon RD, Andrews G, et al. Basic nomenclature issues for DSM-V. In: Kupfer DJ, First MB, Regier DE, editors. A research agenda for DSM-V. Washington, DC: American Psychiatric Association; 2002. p. 1–29.

[4] First MB, Bell CB, Cuthbert B, et al. Personality disorders and relational disorders: a research agenda for addressing critical gaps in DSM. In: Kupfer DJ, First MB, Regier DE, editors. A research agenda for DSM-V. Washington, DC: American Psychiatric Association; 2002. p. 123–99.

[5] Widiger TA, Simonsen E, Krueger R, et al. Personality disorder research agenda for the DSM-V. J Personal Disord 2005;19:317–40.

[6] Oldham JM, Skodol AE. Charting the future of axis II. J Personal Disord 2000;14:17–29.

[7] Widiger TA. Personality disorder dimensional models. In: Widiger TA, Frances AJ, Pincus HA, editors, DSM-IV sourcebook, vol. 2. Washington, DC: American Psychiatric Association; 1996. p. 789–98.

[8] Gunderson JG. DSM-IV personality disorders: final overview. In: Widiger TA, Frances AJ, Pincus HA, editors. DSM-IV sourcebook, vol. 4. Washington, DC: American Psychiatric Association; 1998. p. 1123–40.

[9] Widiger TA, Trull TJ. Plate tectonics in the classification of personality disorder: shifting to a dimensional model. Am Psychol 2007;62:71–83.

[10] Clark LA. Assessment and diagnosis of personality disorder: perennial issues and an emerging reconceptualization. Annu Rev Psychol 2007;58:227–57.

[11] Trull TJ, Durrett CA. Categorical and dimensional models of personality disorder. Annu Rev Clin Psychol 2005;1:355–80.

[12] Widiger TA, Mullins-Sweatt S. Categorical and dimensional models of personality disorder. In: Oldham J, Skodol A, Bender D, editors. Textbook of personality disorders. Washington, DC: American Psychiatric Press; 2005. p. 35–53.

[13] American Psychiatric Association. Diagnostic and statistical manual of mental disorders, 3rd edition, rev ed. Washington, DC: Author; 1987.

[14] Widiger TA, Frances A, Spitzer R, et al. The DSM-III-R personality disorders: an overview. Am J Psychiatry 1988;145:786–95.

[15] Widiger TA, Simonsen E. Alternative dimensional models of personality disorder: finding a common ground. J Personal Disord 2005;19:110–30.

[16] Goldberg LR. The structure of phenotypic personality traits. Am Psychol 1993;48:26–34.

[17] Ashton MC, Lee K. A theoretical basis for the major dimensions of personality. European Journal of Personality 2001;15:327–53.

[18] Costa PT, McCrae RR. Revised NEO personality inventory (NEO PI-R) and NEO five-factor inventory (NEO-FFI) professional manual. Odessa (FL): Psychological Assessment Resources; 1992.

[19] Yamagata S, Suzuki A, Ando J, et al. Is the genetic structure of human personality universal? A cross-cultural twin study from North America, Europe, and Asia. J Pers Soc Psychol 2006;90:987–98.

[20] Schinka JA, Busch RM, Robichaux-Keene N. A meta-analysis of the association between the serotonin transporter gene polymorphism (5-HTTLPR) and trait anxiety. Mol Psychiatry 2004;9(2):197–202.

[21] Sen S, Burmeister M, Ghosh D. Meta-analysis of the association between a serotonin transporter polymorphism (5-HTTLPR) and anxiety-related personality traits. Am J Med Genet 2004;127B:85–9.

[22] Caspi A, Roberts BW, Shiner RL. Personality development: stability and change. Annu Rev Psychol 2005;56:453–84.

[23] Mervielde I, De Clercq B, De Fruyt F, et al. Temperament, personality, and developmental psychopathology as childhood antecedents of personality disorders. J Personal Disord 2005;19:171–201.

[24] Roberts BW, DelVecchio WF. The rank-order consistency of personality traits from childhood to old age: a quantitative review of longitudinal studies. Psychol Bull 2000;126:3–25.

[25] Allik J. Personality dimensions across cultures. J Personal Disord 2005;19:212–32.

[26] Skodol AE, Gunderson JG, Shea MT, et al. The collaborative longitudinal personality disorders study (CLPS): overview and implications. J Personal Disord 2005;19:487–504.

[27] Widiger TA, Costa PT, McCrae RR. A proposal for Axis II: diagnosing personality disorders using the five factor model. In: Costa PT, Widiger TA, editors. Personality disorders and the five factor model of personality. 2nd edition. Washington, DC: American Psychological Association; 2002. p. 431–56.

[28] Mullins-Sweatt SN, Jamerson JE, Samuel SB, et al. Psychometric properties of an abbreviated instrument for the assessment of the five factor model. Assessment 2006;13:119–37.

[29] Mullins-Sweatt SN, Widiger TA. The five-factor model of personality disorder: a translation across science and practice. In: Krueger RF, Tackett JL, editors. Personality and psychopathology. New York: Guilford; 2006. p. 39–70.

[30] Saulsman LM, Page AC. The five-factor model and personality disorder empirical literature: a meta-analytic review. Clin Psychol Rev 2004;23:1055–85.

[31] Widiger TA, Costa PT. Five factor model personality disorder research. In: Costa PT, Widiger TA, editors. Personality disorders and the five factor model of personality. 2nd edition. Washington, DC: American Psychological Association; 2002. p. 59–87.

[32] Widiger TA, Lowe J. Five factor model assessment of personality disorder. J Pers Assess 2007;89:16–29.

[33] Livesley WJ. Conceptual and taxonomic issues. In: Livesley WJ, editor. Handbook of personality disorders. Theory, research, and treatment. New York: Guilford; 2001. p. 3–38.

[34] Clark LA, Simms LJ, Wu KD, et al. Manual for the schedule for nonadaptive and adaptive personality (SNAP-2). Minneapolis (MN): University of Minnesota Press, in press.

[35] Livesley WJ. Diagnostic dilemmas in classifying personality disorder. In: Phillips KA, First MB, Pincus HA, editors. Advancing DSM. Dilemmas in psychiatric diagnosis. Washington, DC: American Psychiatric Association; 2003. p. 153–90.

[36] Samuel DB, Widiger TA. Clinicians' judgments of clinical utility: a comparison of the DSM-IV and five factor models. J Abnorm Psychol 2006;115:298–308.

[37] Lynam DR, Widiger TA. Using the five factor model to represent the DSM-IV personality disorders: an expert consensus approach. J Abnorm Psychol 2001;110:401–12.

[38] Hare RD. Hare psychopathy checklist revised (PCL-R). Technical manual. North Tonawanda (NY): Multi-Health Systems, Inc; 2003.

[39] Cleckley H. The mask of sanity. St. Louis (MO): C.V. Mosby; 1941.

[40] Bell CC. Reservations and hopes. In: Widiger TA, Simonsen E, Sirovatka PJ, editors. Dimensional models of personality disorders. Refining the research agenda for DSM-V. Washington, DC: American Psychiatric Association; 2006. p. 195–8.

[41] Taylor GJ, Bagby RM. New trends in alexithymia research. Psychother Psychosom 2004;73:68–77.

[42] Verheul R. Clinical utility for dimensional models of personality pathology. J Personal Disord 2005;19:283–302.

[43] Maser JD, Kaelber C, Weise RD. International use and attitudes toward DSM-III and DSM-III-R: growing consensus in psychiatric classification. J Abnorm Psychol 1991;100: 271–9.

[44] First MB. Clinical utility: a prerequisite for the adoption of a dimensional approach in DSM. J Abnorm Psychol 2005;114:560–4.

[45] Sartorius N, Schultze H. Reducing the stigma of mental illness. Cambridge (England): Cambridge University Press; 2005.

[46] Millon T, Davis RD, Millon CM, et al. Disorders of personality. DSM-IV and beyond. New York: John Wiley & Sons; 1996.

[47] Sanderson CJ, Clarkin JF. Further use of the NEO PI-R personality dimensions in differential treatment planning. In: Costa PT, Widiger TA, editors. Personality disorders and the five factor model of personality. 2nd edition. Washington, DC: American Psychological Association; 2002. p. 351–75.

[48] American Psychiatric Association. Diagnostic and statistical manual of mental disorders. Text revision. 4th edition. rev. ed. Washington, DC: Author; 2000.

[49] American Psychiatric Association. Practice guidelines for the treatment of patients with borderline personality disorder. Washington, DC: American Psychiatric Association; 2001.

[50] Beck AT, Freeman A, Davis D, et al. Cognitive therapy of personality disorders. 2nd edition. New York: Guilford; 2003.

[51] Derksen J, Maffei C, Groen H, editors. Treatment of personality disorders. Dordrecht (Netherlands): Kluwer Academic Publishers; 1999.

[52] Gunderson JG, Gabbard GO, editors. Psychotherapy for personality disorders. Washington, DC: American Psychiatric Press; 2000.

[53] Livesley WJ. Practical management of personality disorder. New York: Guilford Treatment of personality disorders; 2003.

[54] Paris J. Working with traits: psychotherapy of personality disorders. Lanham (MD): Jason Aronson; 1998.

[55] Paris J. Personality disorders over time: precursors, course, and outcome. Washington, DC: American Psychiatric Publishing; 2003.

[56] Stone MH. Abnormalities of personality. Within and beyond the realm of treatment. New York: W.W. Norton and Company; 1953.

[57] Perry JC, Bond M. Empirical studies of psychotherapy for personality disorders. In: Gunderson JG, Gabbard GO, editors. Psychotherapy for personality disorders. Washington, DC: American Psychiatric Press; 2000. p. 1–31.

[58] Leichsenring F, Leibing E. The effectiveness of psychodynamic therapy and cognitive behavior therapy in the treatment of personality disorders: a meta-analysis. Am J Psychiatry 2003;160: 1223–32.

[59] Linehan M. The empirical basis of dialectical behavior therapy: development of new treatments versus evaluation of existing treatments. Clinical Psychology: Science and Practice 2000;7:113–9.

[60] Scheel KR. The empirical basis of dialectical behavior therapy: summary, critique, and implications. Clinical Psychology: Science and Practice 2000;7:68–86.

The Perils of Dimensionalization: Challenges in Distinguishing Negative Traits from Personality Disorders

Jerome C. Wakefield, PhD, DSW

New York University, Silver School of Social Work, 1 Washington Square North, New York, NY 10003, USA

A major, perhaps dominant trend in the literature on personality disorder (PD) is toward dimensionalization of PD diagnosis in the *Diagnostic and Statistical Manual of Mental Disorders, fifth edition* (DSM-V), where PD will be understood in terms of extreme personality trait dimensions, and thus PD theory will be subsumed under personality-trait theory [1–6]. The basic idea is that extreme traits that lie very high or very low on various personality dimensions–or various combinations of such extreme traits–constitute potential disorders. PD can be diagnosed, according to the usual dimensional approach, when such extreme traits are sufficiently negative and undesirable, as indicated by their being maladaptive, role-impairing, and/or clinically significant [7,8]. In other words, according to the most common dimensional approach, PDs are conceptualized as harmful statistically deviant personality traits.

Yet negative statistically deviant traits are not in general conceptually equivalent to disorders [9]. It appears that nearly everyone has some extreme personality traits–that is, traits that fall very high or very low on some personality dimensions representing degrees of the relevant kind of trait, where the degrees of the trait are often normally distributed in the population–that are negative in at least some situations. Are we then to classify nearly everyone as having PDs under the dimensional proposal? This might be the implication. For example, Thomas Widiger, a leading exponent of a dimensional approach to PD diagnosis, in defending the five-factor model of personality as a basis for an account of PDs as maladaptive traits, observes that "there may be no patient who lacks clinically significant maladaptive personality traits," and then a few lines later puts forward a proposal to diagnose all maladaptive personality traits as PDs: "My recommendation for the diagnosis of personality disorders in future editions of the manual is to recognize explicitly... that personality disorders are maladaptive variants of common personality traits" [10]. Whether intended or

E-mail address: jerome.wakefield@nyu.edu

0193-953X/08/$ – see front matter
doi:10.1016/j.psc.2008.03.009

not, these comments imply that PD may be a universal malady, and that every personality quirk may warrant diagnosis as a personality disorder.

Yet surely the vast majority of people, no matter how irritating they may be at times, do not suffer from PD in the psychiatric sense of a disorder of personality. The problem of defining "caseness" thus poses a serious challenge for the current movement to dimensionalize PD diagnosis in the DSM-V. For, other than an individual's possessing one or more extreme negative personality traits (which, as noted, applies to nearly everyone), it remains unclear how dimensionalized criteria might justifiably warrant the potentially stigmatizing diagnosis of PD and validly distinguish personality disorder from nondisorder.

The problem here is quite different from the general "fuzzy boundary" problem that afflicts most disorder criteria sets. Current DSM criteria for PD do at least try to specify what has gone wrong in the way the overall personality of the individual performs the functions of personality. In contrast, a dimensional approach to diagnosis atomizes the personality into the trait dimensions that are the staple of personality theory. This approach thus loses direct contact with how the traits interact and globally fit together in an overall personality operating within a specific environment. Thus, the potential for false positives goes well beyond the problem of fuzziness at the boundary between disorder and nondisorder and to the heart of what constitutes even a clear case of disorder and nondisorder.

Nor is the problem here the same as the general "clinical significance" problem [11]. Some conditions that technically might satisfy diagnostic criteria are so mild in the intensity of the symptoms that insufficient harm is done to the individual to warrant a diagnosis. Clinical significance requirements—generally, as in the DSM-IV, in the form of significant distress and/or role impairment—attempt to eliminate such mild conditions from the "disorder" category. But the problem with the trait-dimensionalization approach is that it seems that significantly negative traits can still be nondisorders that are part of psychiatrically normal human functioning, analogous to the case of normal grief [12,13].

Sheer statistical extremity of a trait is generally agreed to be an inadequate indicator of disorder; common conditions can be disorders and rare conditions—even rare negative conditions—can be normal [9]. If, as is usually done, the distinction between disorder and nondisorder is made via adding to the extreme negative trait itself some vague additional descriptor such as "maladaptive" or "impairing" or "clinically significant," then the validity problem remains essentially unaddressed, because virtually every negative trait is in some situations maladaptive and impairing of desirable functioning (that's why it's negative!) and thus potentially classifiable as clinically significant. A clinically significant level of impairment that warrants professional intervention does not necessarily represent a disorder, as conditions from marital incompatibility to intense grief illustrate. "Maladaptiveness" has a scientific and even evolutionary ring to it, but it is generally used in the PD literature to refer simply to negative outcomes or social maladjustment, and thus is essentially a value concept that cannot distinguish medical disorder from social undesirability

[14]. So, such descriptors offer no serious progress in distinguishing negative traits from disorders.

Moreover, the idea that statistically extreme traits that are socially maladaptive or impairing are disorders opens the floodgates to use of such diagnoses for social control purposes. In some subcultures, for example, being extremely intelligent or successful in conventional terms may be seen as "selling out" to the dominant culture; thus, within that subculture, these traits are negative, and, due to social ostracism, potentially impairing in certain respects. Does one really want to say that these consequences have anything to do with whether extremely high intelligence or striving for conventional success are disorders, even in that subculture? One thinks here of that wonderful cautionary tale by Kurt Vonnegut that describes a future time when being excellent in any way is taken to be negative because of its unfairness to others and its negative implications for others' self-esteem, and excellence is thus "treated" with various handicaps [15]. It would seem that, by the standard being promulgated by some dimensionalists, we may have to admit that in that future culture, those excellent folks do indeed have a disorder; nor is it clear why the Soviet dissidents might not have been diagnosed with PDs given the proposed approach, given their extreme and surely maladaptive (in their culture) rebelliousness and insistence on the truth and on freedom. One might also ponder here Martin Luther King's admonition that social adjustment to a racist society is not superior mental health.

THE CONFIGURATIONAL, INTEGRATIVE NATURE OF PERSONALITY

The notion that a single problematic trait, or for that matter a set of extreme traits, automatically implies disorder is also inconsistent with the classic conception of personality as a dynamic organization [16]. This conception rejects the notion that personality is sufficiently described by an individual's set of traits, however useful the trait profile might be as an initial assessment and heuristic device. Rather, it is how the overall person incorporates and deals with each of the traits in the social context and within the context of the individual's other traits and intentional states that matters to personality assessment. This view of personality would suggest that a trait profile cannot yield the information necessary for valid diagnosis of PD. The trait profile would always, according to this view, require interpretation in terms of what it means for the overall functioning of the individual. In effect, the trait profile would become a heuristic device preparatory to a diagnosis rather than a diagnostic instrument per se. I believe, but will not try to document here, that ones sees precisely this problem manifested when dimensionalizers try to explain how specific current categories of personality disorders are to be understood in trait profile terms. That is, what you see is a process of interpretation in which an individual's overall personality structure is described so as to make manifest the disorder, but the interpretation is not evident from the trait profile itself. The interpretation explains how the traits fit together within the overall personality to yield a personality disorder, but it is the way the traits interact and what the interaction yields, not anything in the trait profile itself, that constitutes the disorder.

Moreover, I have argued elsewhere that a personality is best thought of not as a set of behaviors or behavioral dispositions, but as a set of basic dispositions to intentional states (ie, mental states such as beliefs, desires, and emotions) that explain behavior [17]. Contrary to approaches to personality in terms of actions, the basic unit of personality consists of the types of mental states one is disposed to have. The "Big Five" factors in the five-factor model of personality can be conceptualized as such motivating internal mental states, with actions often but by no means necessarily correlated. To take a simple example, being high on the trait of "talkative" is not a matter of the high frequency of talking (maybe the individual who talks a lot is an information officer at Penn Station who talks constantly for most of the day; maybe the individual who talks little is in solitary confinement or has his or her jaw wired closed for a lengthy period of time due to a medical condition), nor even of a behavioral disposition to talk (maybe the individual is not naturally talkative but has a deeply unconscious belief that if he or she stops talking other people will dislike him or her and so keeps talking as an instrumental act to avoid anxiety about interpersonal rejection; or maybe the individual is inclined to talk but talks hardly at all because he or she believes that talking is humiliating).

So, if, as I believe must be the case, traits are conceived as theoretical constructs that explain behaviors, then as a matter of the logic of traits, behavior is neither necessary nor sufficient for most personality traits. Consequently, traits can interact with each other and with various intentional states before causing behavior, and unexpected outcomes not captured in a trait assessment may occur due to such interactions. Trying to understand personality as a set of traits with their independent properties is about as hopeless as trying to understand matter as a set of particles with their independent properties; even formation of atoms, let alone molecules, could not be understood in a "particle profile" listing the presence and properties of each type of particle individually.

It is true that, in treating a personality-disordered individual, the clinician tends to focus on and treat specific traits [18–20]. But it is also true that for a diagnosis of PD, one needs to make a global judgment that includes the interaction of various traits, the specific forms of action they give rise to, and the relation of the global configuration to available environmental niches [18–20]. Analogously, once people are judged to be suffering from a depressive disorder, they are often treated for specific symptoms such as blueness or insomnia, but the initial diagnosis of depressive disorder as opposed to normal intense sadness after a loss requires a focus of attention on the context of the symptoms and the nature of the relationship between symptoms and context [13]. Similar issues arise in the diagnosis of conduct disorder [21]; even though once the diagnosis is established, treatment may focus quite narrowly on changing certain behaviors, distinguishing normal delinquency from conduct disorder requires a global assessment with attention to context.

THE FALSE-POSITIVES PROBLEM

Even by current categorical DSM standards, epidemiological surveys indicate that between about a tenth and an eighth of the entire US population has a personality disorder [22,23], already a suspiciously high estimate that suggests some validity problems. If dimensionalization occurs, there is a consequent danger of much more massive numbers of false-positive diagnoses and a general pathologization of the undesirable portions of normal personality variation, leading to much higher rates. But rejection of psychiatric diagnosis as mere medical labeling of undesirable behaviors for purposes of social control, and affirmation of a scientifically based approach that identifies true psychiatric medical disorders and distinguishes them from socially undesirable behaviors, is largely what the modern DSM movement is about. Dimensionalization of personality disorders, then, if done without adequate attention to the false-positives problem—and if, as suggested by some, it serves as a model for what might occur throughout the manual—has the potential to undermine some of the progress that has been made in relegitimizing psychiatry after the disastrous years of the antipsychiatry movement and contributing to the already considerable false-positives problem that afflicts the DSM [24].

Despite these challenges, the problem of how to distinguish negative personality traits from PDs has not been given the conceptual attention it deserves. I have considered the role of cultural variation in judgments about personality disorder in an earlier article [25]. I here undertake to make some further general comments and then to focus on another proposed solution to the problem, the inflexibility criterion.

PERSONALITY DISORDERS FROM THE HARMFUL DYSFUNCTION PERSPECTIVE

My comments here on PD will be broadly from the perspective of the harmful dysfunction (HD) analysis of the concept of mental disorder [26,27]. The HD analysis maintains that a mental disorder is a psychological condition that is negative or harmful according to cultural values and is caused by a dysfunction, that is, by a failure of some psychological mechanism to perform a natural function for which it was biologically designed [28–30]. The HD analysis implies that to achieve a conceptually valid approach to the definition and diagnosis of PD, one must have some idea of what personalities are, why they exist, and what, if anything, personalities are *for* from an evolutionary perspective. Only then can one identify the ways personality can go wrong and fail to perform its functions and thus, if the failure is harmful, be disordered.

From the HD perspective, the reason the "extreme maladaptive trait" approach to defining PD is invalid is easy to see. Maladaptivity, impairment, clinical significance (usually meaning significant distress or role impairment), and other such criteria that are added to statistical abnormality of a trait are essentially "harm" terms, representing social appraisals of negativity. Such harm (which does occur even in the Vonnegut example) is highly sensitive to social values and is necessary but not sufficient for justifiably classifying a condition as a disorder. Even very negative conditions, such as the pain of childbirth, need not be medical disorders.

The other necessary HD criterion for disorder is that there be a dysfunction, that is, that something has gone wrong with biologically designed functioning. In the "extreme maladaptive trait" approach, it is the statistical extremity of the trait along the relevant personality dimension that implicitly attempts to address the dysfunction requirement. However, one of the most basic conceptual findings about mental disorder is that statistical abnormality is not the same as functional abnormality [9]. Statistical extremity can be due to normal variation or it can be due to pathology. But the sheer fact of statistical extremity in and of itself, even in a negative condition, is insufficient for showing that anything has gone wrong. Examples range from normal shortness to normal low intelligence quotient (IQ) to many mental conditions from bad manners to selfishness that are within normal variational parameters but, within our environment and social setting, are negative nonetheless.

If, as appears to be the case, personality traits do vary continuously on trait dimensions, how can an extreme trait (let alone a global configuration into which it enters) ever constitute a dysfunction? At a theoretical level, there are several possibilities, leaving aside global judgments of failure of personality overall to deal with basic life challenges. In exploring these explanatory possibilities, I will use the better understood dimension of intelligence (IQ) as an analogy or model, as have others in the PD literature.

First, the cut-off level may represent a point at which it is inferred that there are likely one or more biological or other specific dysfunctions, independent of the normal distribution itself, that account for the extreme level. For example, the lower extreme end of the intelligence distribution is known to derive in part from over 200 discrete etiological dysfunctions [10]. Second, it may represent a level at which the normal distribution is seen to undermine the function of intelligence itself and, to yield a nonselected level of intelligence that cannot accomplish intelligence's functions (analogous to sickle cell anemia being a chance and unselected end of the random distribution of normal and sickle cell genes that no longer accomplishes the basic functions of the blood). Third, the level of intelligence may be outside the selected range not because it fails to allow success at the specific functions of intelligence but because it has collateral effects that block adequate success in other mechanisms' performance of their functions. That is, the dysfunction lies in how this level of the trait interacts with other traits and their levels.

So, there is a cogent theoretical conception of dysfunction for dimensional variables that is more stringent than social desirability or maladaptiveness within the present environment. At a practical level, as is often the case before an understanding of etiology and underlying mechanisms, only very rough and highly inferential judgments can be made about these properties, but such judgments are implicit in disorder classification.

One might wonder: Why restrict disorder to those conditions that have sources outside the range of biologically selected trait levels? The answer is that the alternative approach undermines the progress psychiatry has made in becoming a medical discipline immune to the typical antipsychiatric criticisms. A basic requirement of such progress is that true medical disorders of the mind be distinguished from socially disapproved conditions (whether or not one chooses to treat the latter). And, the failure of a trait to be within a selected range for that trait dimension can be considered a dysfunction, whereas simply having a negative level of the trait cannot.

Now, it might at first seem acceptable to violate this constraint. Suppose that in primitive environments, the amount of intelligence that was sufficient to confer the fitness benefits of intelligence included IQs from 60 to 70, but the demands of technology, bureaucratic complexity, and multiple options and complex decisions of modern life make an IQ less than 70 insufficient to get along. So, what we have is not a dysfunction but a mismatch between a biologically selected and normal trait and recent changes in the environment. Why not call that a disorder?

However, consider the following thought experiment: imagine that technological advances proceed at such a pace during your lifetime that, just like a generalized version of the Woody Allen character who is simply incapable of figuring out how to get the clock to work on the VCR, your intelligence falls below a new threshold needed to make standard technologies work in an effective manner, so that you can't function effectively in modern society. Does that mean that you and masses of other people now have gotten a disorder, and that more can be given the disorder at will simply by raising the demands of society's technology, or is some other kind of description of what has happened appropriate? The HD analysis suggests the latter answer; biologically designed functioning provides a baseline for judgments of disorder and nondisorder, so social demands are not by themselves determinative of disorder.

WHY EXTREME TRAITS NEED NOT BE PERSONALITY DISORDERS

There are several obstacles to judging disorder on the basis of extreme traits. First, the trait, including at the extreme level, may have been biologically adaptive when selected for, and it may be only in our current rapidly changing environment that the trait is maladaptive. In this case, the organism is biologically and medically normal but is mismatched with the new environment. We may want to intervene with such conditions if they pose problems for social functioning; indeed, I would argue that psychiatry does have as a derived, secondary task the treatment of medically normal conditions that are mismatched with current social values (eg, fear of public speaking, sadness that keeps one from working efficiently, flying phobia) or are just plain undesirable (as in the analogous normal but undesirable physical condition of birth pain).

Why, one might ask, would we not describe such mismatches between human nature as biologically selected and the current social environment as true medical disorders? For one thing, our intuitions in specific cases when the facts are clear go against such classification as pathology. For example, having a taste for fat and sugar appears to be both a naturally selected and originally adaptive disposition under conditions of calorie scarcity yet harmful given our current food-rich environment, but no one considers that a disorder. The fight-or-flight reaction does endless damage both physiologically and interpersonally that is not offset by the benefits in our protected but high stress environments, yet is not a disorder, any more than regrettably high male aggressiveness or unfaithful sexual desires are disorders if indeed they are part of our biologically designed nature, as we believe that they are. But the more basic reason is this: if we were to classify such conditions as disorders, then the category of disorder would cease to have its unusual objective status and could be arbitrarily expanded simply by changing one's social values or environment.

Of course, to adapt to current social demands or opportunities, individuals may want to try to change their psychiatrically normal nature, just as they may want to change their physically normal but unaesthetic appearance. The issue here is how such individuals should be classified, not what they should do. But, how could it be that extreme traits that are judged negative at a substantial enough level that they pass the clinical significance threshold still might be biologically normal? The dimensional approach by its nature judges each dimension separately in the first instance, whereas context goes beyond the five-factor and other models of personality and requires what comes down to a qualitative interpretation of how the individual's various traits integrate into a personality-in-situational-context. So, the context of a trait, generally ignored by the dimensional diagnostic approach except as a transdimensional afterthought, may determine how one should classify it. As a set of suggestive possibilities to ponder in which negative traits do not yield a personality disorder, consider the following:

Negative traits may represent normal variations that were advantageous under other circumstances. If a personality type is no longer desirable because of current cultural values or circumstances, then, rather than the personality type being pathologized as something having gone wrong internally, this situation should be recognized for the mismatch it is, analogous to our reaction to tastes for sugar, fat, and infidelity.

Negative traits may represent personality types selected for their contrast with others and thus for their "niche" within a constellation of competing personality types (eg, conservative versus adventurous, excitable versus stable). Not only is such variation normal, but, for all we know, human culture may be better off with such variety to provide fresh responses when times change.

Negative traits may represent a trade-off for positive traits that is overall useful, where the expansive excellence of one area of functioning is related to the curtailment of excellence in other areas. An example is the reputed trade-off of unusually good spatial-mathematical reasoning ability for a decrease in verbal ability in Einstein's case, and perhaps in others.

Negative traits may be integrated into larger complexes of traits in ways that, although perhaps deviant and provocative, overall are positive or adequately adaptive for the individual. For example, high social anxiety is bad in our high-interaction culture, but throughout history individuals who felt more comfortable working alone intensely on creative projects have benefited themselves and all of us, and certainly need not be judged pathological. Also, despite Peter Kramer's vigorously stated views to the contrary [31], it may be that there is a necessary relationship in some individuals between creativity and depression or even bipolar moods, inasmuch as the pursuit of great goals and the acclaim that may go with them is likely to require persistence through defeats and dismissals that would distress most normal individuals.

Negative traits may represent the lack of suitable niches for the positive expression of the trait under current social circumstances. The social unavailability of adequate niches is thus an alternative hypothesis to PD for some negative traits. For example, forms of fearlessness may be seen as self-threatening and irrational in our current environment, whereas they may be normal, biologically designed variants that were highly useful in the past but have few appropriate niches in our current risk-averse culture. Thus, finding or constructing an appropriate social niche is one route to treating some conditions currently labeled as PDs, especially where personality inappropriateness is due to cultural deprivation of biologically expectable niches for that personality type.

What these types of examples or thought experiments suggest is that the range of psychiatrically normal personality cannot be established by identifying a set of personality dimensions and testing whether any of them are extreme. Rather, a diagnostic assessment must involve evaluation of whether the overall configuration formed as these traits adjust to each other, are shaped by more specific goals and intentional states, and adapt to the social context represents a normal variant, perhaps disadvantaged due to current social demands and values, or a true breakdown in the ability of the personality to serve its basic functions within any of the expectable range of possible social niches.

CONCEPTUAL VALIDITY OF THE INFLEXIBILITY CRITERION

When I recently asked an eminent nosologist how one tells the difference between a negative personality trait and a personality disorder, his answer was immediate: the inflexibility of the trait. This, I think, reflects a common belief in the field by those who recognize that something more is needed to make a trait a disorder than some blanket negative like maladaptiveness (because psychiatrically normal traits can in our environment be maladaptive) or clinical significance (because psychiatrically normal features might be sufficiently distressing or impairing to be significant to the clinician). Inflexibility is one of the most commonly cited of the DSM's general-criteria requirements for personality disorder that could suggest dysfunction. It also has some prima facie plausibility as an indicator of dysfunction, because it has long been an axiom of the mental health field that inflexibility, by narrowing options and precluding adjustment to changing contexts, is potential evidence of disorder.

However, it is not immediately clear how the inflexibility requirement adds to the requirements that a personality trait, and thus a personality disorder, be "enduring" and "pervasive." A condition that is enduring and pervasive is un-varying across time and situations; thus, it might seem, inflexible. For example, the report of the recent National Epidemiologic Survey on Alcohol and Related Conditions [18] defines personality disorders in part as enduring, pervasive, and inflexible. To measure these defining qualities, each respondent was asked regarding each DSM symptom whether the symptom was manifested "most of the time throughout your life, regardless of the situation or who you were with." This question explicitly addresses whether the symptom was enduring and pervasive. Yet it appears to implicitly address inflexibility as well, and it is the only attempt to do so in the survey. So, one might argue that it is poten-tially redundant to add that a pervasive and enduring trait is also inflexible.

One reason for this confusion (and it is a confusion, for inflexibility and pervasiveness are surely different properties) may be that the DSM criteria (and the Survey's questions) are in terms of behavior. Recalling the analysis of personality earlier in this article, traits refer to internal structures that produce internal mental states, and are to be conceptually distinguished from specific behavioral manifestations. Differentiating between traits and their be-havioral expression allows for the needed distinctions. Thus, the trait itself can be enduring (ie, the internal motives are stably generated over many years) and pervasive (ie, the generated motives enter into and influence multiple domains) without being inflexibly behaviorally expressed in those multiple domains. Moreover, inflexibility is a dispositional or capacity concept; a trait is flexible when its expression *would be* adjusted in response to contextual fac-tors *when appropriate*. But capacity is not the same as performance. There can be instances in which traits are expressed in an unvarying, seemingly inflexible manner for appropriate reasons. While behavior should not be confused with the trait that it expresses, I shall argue for the following thesis: it is behavioral inflexibility despite changing situational contexts in instances in which we believe that flexibility of response is part of natural human design that suggests that the trait's expression is contextually unresponsive to a potentially patho-logical degree.

Surely, flexibility, if understood as the capacity to adjust one's response adaptively to the situational context, is a crucial virtue at some times and in some areas of functioning. Yet the suggestion that inflexibility implies dysfunc-tion must be approached with extreme caution. Indeed, another name for what in some contexts might be seen as inflexibility is "integrity." Granting the ideal possibility of a "golden mean," it remains a potential catch-22 to highly value self-cohesiveness as part of health, which demands consistency and overarching strivings that are not subject to the whims of context or "as-if" malleability, and at the same time suggest that flexibility and adaptiveness to context are mea-sures of health.

More importantly, not all psychological mechanisms are designed to be flex-ible, sometimes for good reason. For example, during the 1960s and 1970s, in certain areas of the United States, there arose a view regarding sexual jealousy that painted jealous reactions as born of insecurity or of an oppressive social system and saw them as properly extirpated or at least suppressed. However, those who attempted to flexibly adapt to these changing mores sometimes saw their relationships crumble, whereas those who were less flexible in this regard may have preserved their relationships. Buss's [32] account of sexual jealousy as an essential evolutionarily designed and relatively inflexible mate-guarding and relationship-preserving strategy seems an appropriate antidote to such ideological dismissals of jealousy. Similar cautions might be voiced regarding flexibility in some other areas of personality.

The problem with using inflexibility of personality traits as a basis for attribution of dysfunction can perhaps be appreciated by considering the common analogy of personality traits to IQ. An individual with an IQ of 65 who also meets clinical significance criteria has a presumptive DSM disorder of "mental retardation." Although it is true that this individual's unintelligent thinking is likely to be inflexible across situations, such inflexibility can't be what makes an IQ of 65 a prima facie disorder, because IQ and its expression is rather inflexible across its entire range. The intelligence-related insights of nondisordered individuals with IQs of 100 or 150 are likely to be about equally inflexible across situations as are those of the individual with an IQ of 65. So, whatever it is about an IQ of 65 that makes it a prima facie disorder, it must be something other than inflexible expression of IQ.

The same point holds of many personality traits, whether moderate or extreme. An individual with average empathy may more or less inflexibly experience others' feelings at an average level in all or most empathy-relevant situations, and in this sense be just as "inflexible" in internal trait expression (ie, in generating internal mental states) as an individual with little or no empathy in all situations, or one with very high empathy in all situations. Similarly, an individual who consistently breaks social rules and always places narrow self-interest above cooperation is no more necessarily inflexible than the saintly individual who always thinks in terms of others' needs or the individual who always judges what to do based on a balance of self- and other-needs. Again, it is no more inflexible to be always suspicious of everyone's motives than it is to be always assessing accurately another's motives; true, the latter approach sometimes yields suspicion and sometimes trust as an outcome and thus might be considered more "flexible" in this way, but the internal traits yielding the outcomes are just as inflexible (can a normal individual decide to become paranoid?).

The traditional observation that the psychopath "doesn't learn from experience" may seem to vindicate the inflexibility criterion in this case, but in fact is irrelevant. Personality traits are by definition "enduring," thus inflexible over time and not easily unlearned. High-empathy and high-altruism personalities may not "learn from experience" to be different either, although, like the psychopath, they may as a result of life's lessons learn to be somewhat better at hiding their personal motives and reactions from others.

Indeed, people are often inflexible in their behavior as a matter of choice, principle, or even integrity (ie, being true to their self-perceived ego-syntonic traits). People who "don't suffer fools gladly" may seem inflexible and irritating in their blunt statement of the truth when it would be socially more acceptable and more comfortable to let a foolish comment or a moral lapse pass, yet such inflexibility can be the essence of the person's integrity and their contribution. Consider, for example, the stubborn persistence of Soviet dissidents despite considerable distress and occupational "impairment." Such people, if they become whistle blowers in our society, may lose their jobs, but such "occupational impairment" does not make their (culturally unexpectable) proclivity for the unvarnished truth any more a disorder. Especially once critical periods of social development and identity formation occur, there may be inflexible rigidities in behavior that are normal. For example, throughout history, people have been willing to suffer distress of oppression and even die rather than give up the religion or values into which they were socialized. Was it a disorder for people to maintain their integrity in this inflexible way? We generally consider such a stance to be evidence of the highest form of human courage rather than a disorder, even though it may be inflexible, culturally deviant, and clinically significant (ie, cause a substantial amount of distress or social impairment).

Note also that extremity of a trait in either intensity or frequency of trait expression cannot be equated to the kind of inflexibility supportive of disorder attribution. The individual who is consistently incapable of extreme responses in situations in which they are appropriate is just as relevantly inflexible as the individual who is incapable of moderating responses when appropriate. Moreover, because action issues from an interaction of many traits and meanings, action that is different from that usually implied by a trait does not imply lack of extremes of the trait. The avoidant person who is also highly sociable may sometimes (due to their longing for company) overcome their fears and socialize. To that extent, there is behavioral flexibility yet extremity of the underlying trait.

These cautions notwithstanding, there surely is a kind of inflexibility of a trait that may well support an inference that personality pathology exists. Although many traits by their very nature are inflexible, the behavioral expression of the trait is often designed to be capable of flexibility when overridden by other motives. Consequently, an inability to regulate trait behavioral expression in accordance with context would in some instances suggest a dysfunction. For example, one's sense of humor as a trait may stay the same, but one still ought to be able to control one's natural inclination to laughter when socially inappropriate; similarly, one's empathic sense may stay the same across situations, but whether one expresses empathy should shift according to the social situation. Indeed, even the psychopath may have sufficient flexibility at the behavioral level to follow the rules for awhile if it suits him or her, as when such an individual follows the rules of therapy in search of some benefit from the therapist.

To take another example, some creative people can create at their highest level only under rather specific conditions (eg, open time, isolation), and their lives involve a constant struggle to realize those conditions in the face of objections from intimates who may see the individual's requirements as irritating and perhaps even pathologically inflexible. In reality, the individual has to be assertive and rather uncompromising in arranging his or her life to allow for the creative conditions to be realized simply as an instrumental strategy for optimal achievement and self-realization given their mental nature and the constraints of the environment. Of course, it would be better if creative intellectuals and artists were more flexible and could work under whatever conditions happen to exist, and, enviably, many are; but others are not, and there is nothing necessarily pathological about such inflexibility in trying to derive the most from their gifts.

The example of creativity suggests the broader problem that even extreme and rigid traits can be highly useful in specific social roles. If the diversity of personality is partly designed to allow individuals to adapt to varying social niches, then imposing one ideal template on all individuals would be a mistake. For example, the behaviors associated with DSM-IV obsessive-compulsive personality disorder were found in a recent survey to be only weakly associated with reports of social or personal disability [22], and one reason may be that the American workplace is an environment in which the behaviors associated with this presumed personality disorder can be highly adaptive and rewarding. Perhaps this is merely the finding of a niche where a dysfunction does no harm; or perhaps there is no dysfunction at all but only normal variation in the first place. But what is clear is that, because of the requirement that a dysfunction must cause significant harm if it is to labeled a disorder, social opportunities for using extreme traits constructively may determine whether a condition is a disorder, and inflexibility becomes irrelevant.

Personality disorder thus represents a breakdown in the central function of personality, namely, as an emergent organization that integrates traits and other mental states and mechanisms to accomplish basic tasks. To put it in cognitive terms, the dysfunction, according to this view of inflexibility, is the fact that there is a breakdown in normal penetrability of trait expression by alternative motives. In psychodynamic terms, it is a failure of integration. In evolutionary terms, it is a failure of functional hierarchical organization in which each trait's expression is subject to regulation by the overall personality organization.

The inclination to be polite is not necessarily any more or less flexible than the inclination to be abrasive or obsequious (Michael Stone considers the latter extremes pathological [33]); the polite person feels uncomfortable being abrasive or obsequious and generally sticks to the middle road. Thus, the danger of the "inflexibility" requirement is that it is hiding the true and highly value-determined nature of the diagnostic process, which is that the criteria are applied only to those traits that we do not like. That is, by "inflexible" we could implicitly mean that the trait is one of which we disapprove but that the individual cannot or will not change nonetheless. It is, in other words, a tool of social control: the consistently criminal individual is inflexible in his or her behavior because of being unable to change toward social norms, justifying our intervention; but the equally consistently law-abiding person is merely considered reasonable and moral.

What all of this suggests is that the "inflexibility" requirement is a misdirected way of trying to say something else. I think what it is trying to say is this: A personality disorder exists when there is a malfunction of personality organization, and one possible indicator of such a malfunction is that there is a trait that is pathologically inflexible in the sense that it is designed to be situationally sensitive and/or to be behaviorally flexible in response to internal and external context, but the individual lacks the designed capacity to modulate and regulate the expression of the trait in response to competing traits, situational context, or the overall dictates of reason.

I conclude that it is neither inflexibility of a trait per se (for that is often normally the case), nor inflexibility of behavior per se (for that may be either a matter of instrumental strategy or situational response), that may imply personality disorder (when cultural-deviance and clinical-significance criteria are met). Rather, disorder is indicated by the inability of the overall personality to incorporate that inflexibility into an adequate solution to life tasks, in cases where flexibility seems a design feature of the motivational system and where the environment includes an expectable range of niches from which the individual may choose. Thus, inflexibility suggests disorder only when it suggests failure of biological design.

References

[1] Costa PT, Widiger TA. Personality disorders and the five-factor model of personality. 2nd edition. Washington, DC: American Psychological Association; 2002.

[2] Widiger TA, Costa PT. Personality and personality disorders. J Abnorm Psychol 1994;103: 78–91.

[3] Widiger TA, Lowe JR. Five-factor model assessment of personality disorder. J Pers Assess 2007;89:16–29.

[4] Widiger TA, Simonson E. Alternative dimensional models of personality disorder: finding a common ground. J Personal Disord 2005;19:110–30.

[5] Widiger TA, Simonsen E, Krueger R, et al. Personality disorder research agenda for the DSM–V. J Personal Disord 2005;19:315–38.

[6] Widiger TA, Trull TJ. Plate tectonics in the classification of personality disorder: shifting to a dimensional model. Am Psychol 2007;62:71–83.

[7] Widiger TA, Costa PT, McCrae RR. A proposal for axis II: diagnosing personality disorders using the five factor model. In: Costa PT, Widiger TA, editors. Personality disorders and the five-factor model of personality. 2nd edition. Washington, DC: American Psychological Association; 2002. p. 431–56.

[8] Widiger TA, Lowe JR. A dimensional model of personality disorder: proposal for DSM-V. Psychiatr Clin North Am 2008;31:363–78.

[9] Wakefield JC. The concept of mental disorder: on the boundary between biological facts and social values. Am Psychol 1992;47:373–88.

[10] Widiger TA. Personality disorders in the 21st century. J Personal Disord 2000;14:3–16.

[11] Spitzer RL, Wakefield JC. DSM-IV diagnostic criterion for clinical significance: Does it help solve the false positives problem? Am J Psychiatry 1999;156:1856–64.

[12] Wakefield JC, Schmitz MF, First MB, et al. Should the bereavement exclusion for major depression be extended to other losses? Evidence from the national comorbidity survey. Arch Gen Psychiatry 2007;64:433–40.

[13] Horwitz AV, Wakefield JC. The loss of sadness: how psychiatry transformed normal sorrow into depressive disorder. New York: Oxford University Press; 2007.

[14] Clark LA. Evaluation and devaluation in personality assessment. In: Sadler JZ, editor. Descriptions & prescriptions: values, mental disorders, and the DSMs. Baltimore (MD): John Hopkins University Press; 2002. p. 131–47.

[15] Vonnegut K. Harrison Bergeron. In Welcome to the monkey house. New York: Delacorte; 1968. p. 7–14.

[16] Allport GW. Pattern and growth in personality. New York: Holt, Rinehart, Winston; 1961.

[17] Wakefield JC. Levels of explanation in personality theory. In: Buss D, Cantor N, editors. Personality psychology: recent trends and emerging directions. New York: Springer-Verlag; 1989. p. 333–46.

[18] Paris J. Working with traits: psychotherapy of personality disorders. Lanham (MD): Jason Aronson; 1998.

[19] Paris J. Personality disorders over time: precursors, course, and outcome. Washington, DC: American Psychiatric Publishing; 2003.

[20] Paris J. Social factors in the personality disorders: a biopsychosocial approach to etiology and treatment. Cambridge (UK): Cambridge University Press; 1994.

[21] Wakefield JC, Pottick KJ, Kirk SA. Should the DSM-IV diagnostic criteria for conduct disorder consider social context? Am J Psychiatry 2002;159:380–6.

[22] Grant BF, Hasin DS, Stinson FS, et al. Prevalence, correlates, and disability of personality disorders in the U.S.: results from the national epidemiologic survey on alcohol and related conditions. J Clin Psychiatry 2004;65:948–58.

[23] Lenzenweger MF, Lane MC, Loranger AW, et al. DSM-IV personality disorders in the National Comorbidity Survey Replication. Biol Psychiatry 2007;62:553–64.

[24] Wakefield JC. Diagnosing DSM-IV, part 1: DSM-IV and the concept of mental disorder. Behav Res Ther 1997;35:633–50.

[25] Wakefield JC. Personality disorder as harmful dysfunction: DSM's cultural deviance requirement reconsidered. J Personal Disord 2006;20:157–69.

[26] Wakefield JC. Disorder as harmful dysfunction: a conceptual critique of DSM-III-R's definition of mental disorder. Psychol Rev 1992;99:232–47.

[27] Wakefield JC. Limits of operationalization: a critique of Spitzer and Endicott's (1978) proposed operational criteria for mental disorder. J Abnorm Psychol 1993;102:160–72.

[28] Wakefield JC. Evolutionary versus prototype analyses of the concept of disorder. J Abnorm Psychol 1999;108:374–99.

[29] Livesley WJ. Conceptual and taxonomic issues. In: Livesley WJ, editor. Handbook of personality disorders. New York: Guilford; 2001. p. 3–38.

[30] Livesley WJ, Schroeder ML, Jackson DN, et al. Categorical distinctions in the study of personality disorder: implications for classification. J Abnorm Psychol 1994;108:374–99.

[31] Kramer PD. Against depression. New York: Penguin; 2005.

[32] Buss DM. The dangerous passion: why jealousy is as necessary as love and sex. New York: The Free Press; 2000.

[33] Stone MH. Treatment of personality disorders from the perspective of the five-factor model. In: Costa PT, Widiger TA, editors. Personality disorders and the five-factor model of personality. 2nd edition. Washington, DC: American Psychological Association; 2002. p. 405–30.

Epidemiology of Personality Disorders

Mark F. Lenzenweger, PhD[a,b,*]

[a]Department of Psychology, State University of New York at Binghamton, Binghamton, NY, USA
[b]Department of Psychiatry, Weill Medical College of Cornell University, New York, NY, USA

The prevalence of personality disorder (PD) in the nonclinical (community) population was largely unknown through the early 1990s, although it was of considerable interest to the architects of the *Diagnostic and Statistical Manual of Mental Disorders* (DSM) system, the National Institute of Mental Health (NIMH), and the personality disorders research community. The prevalence estimates provided in the DSM manuals (DSM-III, DSM-III-R, DSM-IV) were essentially informed speculation, but they did not derive from properly designed population studies. Some specific disorders, such as borderline PD, were simply described as "common" [1–3]. At the NIMH-sponsored workshop on personality disorders held at Williamsburg, VA, in 1990, Weissman [4] conjectured that the population prevalence of "any PD" would be in the range of 10% to 13%. The "guess-timate" informed by early (1950s) community surveys and the rate of PDs observed in the biological relatives of psychopathology-affected subjects who were participating in other studies (eg, the nonpsychotic relatives of schizophrenia patients; or, healthy control subjects and their biological relatives). Clearly, this prior database was subject to a variety of methodological artifacts. For example, the early community studies did not use explicit diagnostic criteria for the definition of PD, nor could they have used structured interviews, as they did not exist in the 1950s. The study of the rate of PD in the relatives of psychiatric patients (eg, first-degree relatives of psychotic patients) resulted in data hampered by the fact that the samples were necessarily conditioned on the presence of major psychotic symptomatology in the study probands as well as the fact that biological relationships among the study subjects precluded independence of observation across the samples. In short, the sample selection and relatedness of the subjects shaped the samples in ways that would not be characteristic of samples drawn from the population at large. Thus, issues of diagnosis, sampling, and disorder definition loomed large in the consideration of data drawn from these early studies. Nonetheless, the

Preparation of this review was supported by sabbatical funds from the State University of New York at Binghamton.

*Department of Psychology, State University of New York at Binghamton, Science IV, Binghamton, NY 13902. *E-mail address*: mlenzen@binghamton.edu

0193-953X/08/$ – see front matter
doi:10.1016/j.psc.2008.03.003

"guess-timate" conjectured by Weissman [4] provided an initial starting value to consider when evaluating the results of subsequent community-based studies.

Clearly, community-based studies were needed to provide a proper estimate for PD prevalence in the general population. Prevalence rates simply could not be estimated from biased samples recruited for other studies. Nor could they be effectively estimated from the study of consecutive admissions to psychiatric hospitals and/or clinics. Simply put, it was not known whether PD patients presenting at clinics and hospital settings were representative of the population of PD-affected individuals. However, in light of what was known about *Berkson's Bias* [5] in the epidemiology literature, it seemed highly likely that clinic/hospital patients would not only be unrepresentative of the population of PD-affected cases (eg, showing more severe PD impairment, perhaps greater Axis II comorbidity), but they would also likely present with greater pathology of all sorts (eg, Axis I, medical disorders, and other impairment). Moreover, some PD patients might be less likely to present at clinics unless they were in a state of crisis, for example, schizotypal or paranoid PD patients.

It is well known from the clinical literature that PDs are highly comorbid with a wide range of Axis I disorders [6–11], that the impairment in role functioning due to PDs is substantial [12–14], and that people with PDs are heavy users of both primary care and mental health services [14–17]. Thus, accurate community-based prevalence estimates have long been sought after given their obvious utility for public health planning matters as well as basic scientific research.

THE LONGITUDINAL STUDY OF PERSONALITY DISORDERS: AN INITIAL ESTIMATE

A sea change in the epidemiology of the PDs began in the early 1990s with the inception of the *Longitudinal Study of Personality Disorders* (LSPD) [18], the first NIMH-sponsored longitudinal study of personality pathology. The LSPD was undertaken in a nonclinical population from which study samples were drawn for long-term prospective study of PD, personality, and temperament. The LSPD used a two-stage selection procedure for the selection of study subjects for the planned longitudinal investigation. In short, a nonclinical university population (n = 2000) was sampled in a representative fashion and screened with a psychometric screen for personality disorder known as the *International Personality Disorder Examination-Screen* (IPDE-S), developed in the context of developing the *International Personality Disorder Examination* [19,20]. The overall sample was parsed as a function of those who screened positive for a personality disorder versus those who did not. Subsamples of those who screened PD-positive or PD-negative were subsequently interviewed using the IPDE. This provided a novel opportunity to employ the powerful two-stage approach to case identification [21] for the generation of a prevalence estimate for personality pathology in a nonclinical population. Lenzenweger and colleagues [22] reported a point prevalence of 11.01% (95% CI 7.57%–14.52%) for "any PD." This figure accounted not only for specific PD diagnoses (definite + probable cases), but also included the category PD Not Otherwise Specified (PD-NOS). The breakdown for prevalence rates for specific PDs and DSM-III-R cluster PD (Cluster A "odd, eccentric," Cluster B "erratic, impulsive," Cluster C "anxious, avoidant") in the LSPD can be seen in Table 1.

INTERNATIONAL STUDIES OF PERSONALITY DISORDER PREVALENCE

Torgersen and colleagues [23] conducted an epidemiologic study of PD in Oslo, Norway, in a representative sample of 2053 adults between the ages of 18 and 65. Using the Structured Interview for DSM-III-R Personality Disorders (SIDP-R) [24] administered by experienced psychiatric nurses, Torgersen and colleagues [23] found a prevalence for "any PD" of 13.4% (weighted %). In their sample, Cluster C disorders appeared to be more common (9.4%) than either Cluster A (4.1%) or Cluster B (3.1%). No sex differences were found at the level of any of the three PD clusters.

Coid and colleagues [25] conducted a national survey of PD in Great Britain among adults using a two-stage procedure for case identification. The first-stage Axis II screening was conducted within the British National Survey of Psychiatric Morbidity and included 8886 subjects (69.5% response rate). Subjects were selected for assessment at the second stage on the basis of their PD status as determined in the first-stage screening. The second-stage assessments (n = 638) were conducted on those agreeing to participate using the Structured Clinical Interview for DSM-IV Axis II Disorders (SCID-II) [26] interview. Coid and colleagues [25] found an overall prevalence rate of 10.1% for "any PD" (including PD-NOS) and they also reported rates for specific PDs as well as the PD clusters (see Table 1). The rates of Cluster A, B, and C PDs were all broadly comparable; the most frequent diagnosis in the Coid and colleagues [25] study was PD-NOS (5.7%). Cluster B PDs, but not Cluster A or Cluster C PDs, were significantly more common in women than men.

COMMUNITY STUDIES IN THE UNITED STATES

Samuels and colleagues [27] reported PD prevalence rates for one of the original sites in the well-known Epidemiologic Catchment Area Study, specifically the Baltimore, MD, site. In a sample of 742 adults (ages 34 to 94), Samuels and colleagues [27] used the IPDE, administered by experienced clinical psychologists, and found an overall prevalence rate of 9.0% for "any personality disorder." Their sample was noteworthy for a high rate of antisocial personality disorder (4.1%), which led to a somewhat higher rate of Cluster B PDs relative to Cluster A and C PDs. Cluster A and B, but not Cluster C, disorders were found to be significantly more common in men than women.

Crawford and colleagues [28], reporting from the *Children in the Community Study* (directed by Patricia Cohen, PhD), found in a sample of 644 adults (average age = 33 years) that 15.7% of their sample had some form of PD. The Axis II diagnostic assessments were conducted by clinically experienced

Table 1
The prevalence (percentage) of personality disorders in six nonclinical population/community studies using validated structured interviews

	Study					
	Lenzenweger et al [22]	Torgersen et al [23]	Samuels et al [27]	Crawford et al [28][a]	Coid et al [25]	Lenzenweger et al [30]
Instrument	IPDE	SIDP-R	IPDE[b]	SCID-II	SCID-II	IPDE
Nomenclature	DSM-III-R	DSM-III-R	DSM-IV	DSM-IV	DSM-IV	DSM-IV
Location	Ithaca, NY, USA	Oslo, Norway	Baltimore, MD, USA	Upstate New York, USA	Great Britain [National]	United States [National]
Personality Disorder						
Paranoid	1.0	2.4	0.7	5.1	.7	—
Schizoid	1.0	1.7	0.9	1.7	.8	—
Schizotypal	1.6	0.6	0.6	1.1	.06	—
Cluster A	2.8	4.1	2.1	6.8	1.6	5.7
Antisocial	0.6	0.7	4.1	1.2	.6	.6
Borderline	1.3	0.7	0.5	3.9	.7	1.4
Histrionic	2.9	2.0	0.2	.9	—	—
Narcissistic	2.7	0.8	0.03	2.2	—	—
Cluster B	5.3	3.1	4.5	6.1	1.2	1.5

Avoidant	1.0	5.0	1.8	6.4	.8	—
Dependent	0.6	1.5	0.1	.8	.1	—
Obsessive-Compulsive	1.3	2.0	—	4.7	1.9	—
Passive-Aggressive	1.6	1.7	—	—	—	—
Cluster C	2.6	9.4[d]	2.8	10.6	1.6	6.0
Any PD	11.01[c]	13.4[d]	9.0	15.7	10.1[e]	9.1[f]

Instruments indicate the structured clinical interview used: International Personality Disorder Examination (IPDE); Structured Interview for DSM-III-R Personality Disorders (SIDP-R); Structured Clinical Interview for DSM-IV Axis II Disorders (SCID-II). Dashes indicate not applicable. All prevalences reported are weighted prevalences.

Abbreviations: DSM, Diagnostic and Statistical Manual of Mental Disorders; PD, personality disorder.

[a] Prevalences for antisocial PD and histrionic PD were estimated using self-report data [28].

[b] IPDE (DSM-IV version) [19].

[c] Includes sadistic PD as well as PD–Not Otherwise Specified (PD-NOS) based on the IPDE (DSM-III-R version).

[d] Includes self-defeating, fearful, and sadistic PDs.

[e] Includes PD-NOS.

[f] Includes PD-NOS. All National Comorbidity Survey Replication (NCS-R) prevalence rates are based on multiply imputed values in nationally representative sample of subjects from the United States. See Lenzenweger and colleagues [30] for extensive technical detail.

staff using the SCID-II interview. These authors found Cluster A and Cluster B PD prevalence rates to be broadly comparable (6.8% and 6.1% respectively), whereas Cluster C PDs were somewhat more prevalent (10.6%). Sex differences were not reported in Crawford and colleagues [28].

A NATIONALLY REPRESENTATIVE STUDY IN THE UNITED STATES: NATIONAL COMORBIDITY SURVEY REPLICATION

Each of the prior studies done in the United States focused on samples drawn from populations possessing unique characteristics (eg, university students; inner city Baltimore, MD; rural Upstate New York) that potentially limited their results in terms of generalizability to the United States as a whole. Thus, it was decided to address this gap in the psychiatric epidemiology of the United States within the context of the *National Comorbidity Survey Replication* (NCS-R) [29]. It was deemed essential to have clinically experienced diagnosticians using a well-validated structured clinical interview conduct the assessments for the NCS-R. Clearly, all members of the representative national sample drawn for the NCS-R (n > 5000) could not be interviewed face-to-face for the Axis II assessments. Therefore, it was decided to employ the two-stage procedure for case identification and a screen would be used in the preliminary assessment phase of the NCS-R. Given that the IPDE-Screen had performed very well in the LSPD [29], it was selected for inclusion in the NCS-R. Specifically, there were no cases of "definite" PD associated with a positive IPDE-S screening value (ie, no false negatives) in the LSPD. The second-stage Axis II assessments conducted for the NCS-R were done using the IPDE. A complex multiple imputation procedure was then used to estimate population prevalences for PDs from the clinical reappraisal sample (second-stage assessment sample) for the sample as a whole (see Lenzenweger and colleagues [30] for extensive technical detail). As can be seen in Table 1, the overall prevalence rate for PD in the US population was found to be 9% [30]. A noteworthy feature of the NCS-R PD data was the estimation of prevalence rates for specific Cluster B PDs, namely borderline and antisocial PDs. Borderline PD was found to have a general population prevalence of 1.4%, whereas antisocial PD had a prevalence of 0.6%. The NCS-R PD prevalence rates were not associated with sex at the level of clusters or "any PD"; however, there was a nontrivial trend for antisocial PD to be less prevalent in women. Of particular note, borderline personality disorder was equally common in men and women. Finally, as found in many prior inpatient and outpatient samples, a wide range of Axis I disorders were frequently comorbid with the Axis II disorders diagnosed in the NCS-R subjects (across all three PD clusters) [30].

In this context, I note that a study by Grant and colleagues [31] also sought to estimate prevalence rates for a subset of Axis II disorders using a national population sample. However, the data from this study are not discussed here as that study did not use a validated Axis II diagnostic instrument and the Axis II assessments were done by census workers with minimal experience in the diagnosis of severe psychopathology.

SUMMARY

These modern epidemiological studies, each conducted in different populations, yield remarkably consistent estimates for "any PD" as defined by the DSM system and assessed using a validated structured clinical interview in the hands of experienced diagnosticians. The median prevalence rate for "any PD" across these studies is 10.56% and the mean prevalence rate is 11.39%. Despite variation in methods and instrumentation, these data indicate that approximately 1 in every 10 persons suffers from a diagnosable personality disorder. Personality pathology is clearly a frequently occurring phenomenon and a matter for concern from the standpoint of public health (ie, treatment use, impact on occupational functioning). Sex differences do not appear to have a consistent pattern for the PDs across the various studies. These studies also highlight the utility of the PD-NOS diagnosis, which was found to be relatively common in several studies (eg, see Lenzenweger and colleagues [22] and Coid and colleagues [25]). Finally, from the standpoint of research, the relatively high rate of PD serves as a powerful stimulus for efforts to understand the neurobiology of PD [32,33], resolve endophenotypes for the specific PDs [34,35], illuminate issues of stability and change in PDs across the lifespan [36,37], and determine which are the most effective treatments for PD [38].

References

[1] American Psychiatric Association. Diagnostic and statistical manual of mental disorders (DSM-III). 3rd edition. Washington, DC: American Psychiatric Association; 1980.

[2] American Psychiatric Association. Diagnostic and statistical manual of mental disorders (DSM-III-R). 3rd edition–revised. Washington, DC: American Psychiatric Association; 1987.

[3] American Psychiatric Association. Diagnostic and statistical manual of mental disorders (DSM-IV). 4th edition. Washington, DC: American Psychiatric Association; 1994.

[4] Weissman MM. The epidemiology of personality disorders: a 1990 update. J Personal Disord 1993;7:44–62.

[5] Berkson J. Limitations of the application of fourfold table analysis to hospital data. Biometrics 1946;2:339–43.

[6] Goodwin RD, Brook JS, Cohen P. Panic attacks and the risk of personality disorder. Psychol Med 2005;35:227–35.

[7] Johnson JG, Cohen P, Kasen S, et al. Personality disorder traits associated with risk for unipolar depression during middle adulthood. Psychiatry Res 2005;136:113–21.

[8] Loranger AW. The impact of DSM-III on diagnostic practice in a university hospital. A comparison of DSM-II and DSM-III in 10,914 patients. Arch Gen Psychiatry 1990;47: 672–5.

[9] Mattia JI, Zimmerman M. Epidemiology. In: Livesley WJ, editor. Handbook of personality disorders: theory, research, and treatment. New York: The Guilford Press; 2001. p. 107–23.

[10] McGlashan TH, Grilo CM, Skodol AE, et al. The collaborative longitudinal personality disorders study: baseline axis I/II and II/II diagnostic co-occurrence. Acta Psychiatr Scand 2000;102:256–64.

[11] Oldham JM, Skodol AE, Kellman HD, et al. Comorbidity of axis I and axis II disorders. Am J Psychiatry 1995;152:571–8.

[12] Johnson JG, First MB, Cohen P, et al. Adverse outcomes associated with personality disorder not otherwise specified in a community sample. Am J Psychiatry 2005;162:1926–32.

[13] Keel PK, Dorer DJ, Eddy KT, et al. Predictors of treatment utilization among women with anorexia and bulimia nervosa. Am J Psychiatry 2002;159:140–2.

[14] Miller JD, Pilkonis PA, Mulvey EP. Treatment utilization and satisfaction: examining the contributions of axis II psychopathology and the five-factor model of personality. J Personal Disord 2006;20:369–87.

[15] Skodol AE, Gunderson JG, McGlashan TH, et al. Functional impairment in patients with schizotypal, borderline, avoidant, or obsessive-compulsive personality disorder. Am J Psychiatry 2002;159:276–83.

[16] Bender DS, Dolan RT, Skodol AE, et al. Treatment utilization by patients with personality disorders. Am J Psychiatry 2001;158:295–302.

[17] Moran P, Rendu A, Jenkins R, et al. The impact of personality disorder in UK primary care: a 1-year follow-up of attenders. Psychol Med 2001;31:1447–54.

[18] Lenzenweger MF. The longitudinal study of personality disorders: history, design, and initial findings [special essay]. J Personal Disord 2006;6:645–70.

[19] Loranger AW. International personality disorder examination: DSM-IV and ICD-10 interviews. Odessa (FL): Psychological Assessment Resources, Inc; 1999.

[20] Loranger AW, Sartorius N, Andreoli A, et al. The international personality disorder examination (IPDE). The world health organization/alcohol, drug abuse, and mental health administration international pilot study of personality disorders. Arch Gen Psychiatry 1994;51:215–24.

[21] Shrout P, Newman SC. Design of two-phase prevalence studies of rare disorders. Biometrics 1989;45:549–55.

[22] Lenzenweger MF, Loranger AW, Korfine L, et al. Detecting personality disorders in a non-clinical population. Application of a 2-stage procedure for case identification. Arch Gen Psychiatry 1997;54:345–51.

[23] Torgersen S, Kringlen E, Cramer V. The prevalence of personality disorders in a community sample. Arch Gen Psychiatry 2001;58:590–6.

[24] Pfohl B, Blum N, Zimmerman M. Structured interview for DSM-IV personality (SIDP-IV). Washington, DC: American Psychiatric Press, Inc; 1997.

[25] Coid J, Yang M, Tyrer P, et al. Prevalence and correlates of personality disorder among adults aged 16 to 74 in Great Britain. Br J Psychiatry 2006;188:423–31.

[26] First MB, Gibbon M, Spitzer RL, et al. Structured clinical interview for DSM-IV axis II personality disorders (SCID-II), version 2.0. New York: Biometrics Research Department, New York State Psychiatric Institute; 1994.

[27] Samuels J, Eaton WW, Bienvenu OJ III, et al. Prevalence and correlates of personality disorders in a community sample. Br J Psychiatry 2002;180:536–42.

[28] Crawford TN, Cohen P, Johnson JG, et al. Self-reported personality disorder in the children in the community sample: convergent and prospective validity in late adolescence and adulthood. J Personal Disord 2005;19:30–52.

[29] Kessler RC, Berglund P, Chiu WT, et al. The US National Comorbidity Survey Replication (NCS-R): design and field procedures. Int J Methods Psychiatr Res 2004;13:69–92.

[30] Lenzenweger MF, Lane M, Loranger AW, et al. DSM-IV personality disorders in the National Comorbidity Survey Replication (NCS-R). Biol Psychiatry 2007;62:553–64.

[31] Grant BF, Hasin DS, Stinson FS, et al. Prevalence, correlates, and disability of personality disorders in the United States: results from the national epidemiologic survey on alcohol and related conditions. J Clin Psychiatry 2004;65:948–58.

[32] Depue RA, Lenzenweger MF. A neurobehavioral model of personality disturbance. In: Clarkin JF, Lenzenweger MF, editors. Major theories of personality disorder. 2nd edition. New York: Guilford; 2005. p. 391–453.

[33] Lenzenweger MF, Clarkin JF. The personality disorders: history, development, and research issues. In: Clarkin JF, Lenzenweger MF, editors. Major theories of personality disorder. 2nd edition. New York: Guilford Press; 2005. p. 1–42.

[34] Lenzenweger MF, Clarkin JF, Fertuck EA, et al. Executive neurocognitive functioning and neurobehavioral systems indicators in borderline personality disorder: a preliminary study. J Personal Disord 2004;18:421–38.

[35] Silbersweig D, Clarkin JF, Goldstein M, et al. Failure of the fronto-limbic inhibitory function in the context of negative emotion in borderline personality disorder. Am J Psychiatry 2007;164:1832–41.

[36] Lenzenweger MF, Johnson MD, Willett JB. Individual growth curve analysis illuminates stability and change in personality disorder features: the longitudinal study of personality disorders. Arch Gen Psychiatry 2004;61:1015–24.

[37] Lenzenweger MF, Willett JB. Modeling individual change in personality disorder features as a function of simultaneous individual change in personality dimensions linked to neurobehavioral systems: the longitudinal study of personality disorders. J Abnorm Psychol 2007;116: 684–700.

[38] Clarkin JF, Levy KN, Lenzenweger MF, et al. Evaluating three treatments for borderline personality disorder: a multiwave study. Am J Psychiatry 2007;164:922–8.

The Frequency of Personality Disorders in Psychiatric Patients

Mark Zimmerman, MD*, Iwona Chelminski, PhD,
Diane Young, PhD

Department of Psychiatry and Human Behavior, Brown University School of Medicine, Rhode
Island Hospital, Bayside Medical Center, 235 Plain Street, Providence, RI 02905, USA

C ommunity-based epidemiological studies of psychiatric disorders provide important information about the public health burden of these
problems. While the frequency of treatment-seeking for psychiatric disorders may be increasing [1], epidemiological studies indicate that most patients
in the community do not get treatment for psychiatric disorders [2,3]. Seeking
treatment is related to a number of clinical and demographic factors [4,5]; consequently, studies of the frequency and correlates of psychiatric disorders in the
general population should be replicated in clinical populations to provide the
practicing clinician with information that might have more direct clinical utility.

Differences between general population and clinical epidemiological studies
might be greatest when examining disorder prevalence and diagnostic comorbidity. It is not appropriate to extrapolate from community-based prevalence
rates to clinical settings where the disorder rates are higher. Comorbidity rates
are also expected to be higher in clinical settings because help seeking is related
to comorbidity [6].

Diagnosing co-occuring personality disorders in psychiatric patients with an
Axis I disorder is clinically important because of their association with the duration, recurrence, and outcome of Axis I disorders [7–9]. Differential diagnosis
amongst the personality disorders has implications for psychotherapeutic and
pharmacologic approaches [10]. An Axis II diagnosis, similar to an Axis I
diagnosis, succinctly communicates important clinical information from one
clinician to another. In addition to clinicians benefiting from such communication, patients may also benefit in a therapeutic fashion following being informed that they meet criteria for an Axis II diagnosis [11].

METHODOLOGICAL CONSIDERATIONS IN THE ASSESSMENT OF PERSONALITY DISORDERS

The who, what, when, and how of assessment can influence the results of a
clinical epidemiological study.

*Corresponding author. E-mail address: mzimmerman@lifespan.org (M. Zimmerman).

0193-953X/08/$ – see front matter
doi:10.1016/j.psc.2008.03.015

Who Should be Interviewed—the Patient, an Informant, or Both?

Research on the respective validity of different sources of information is sparse. However, some studies have found that when information from informants is ascertained to supplement patient information, then the prevalence rates increase [12].

When Should Personality Disorders be Assessed?

The reason for even asking this question is because of the well-known effect of psychiatric state on personality assessment. Acute psychiatric state can inflate personality disorder estimates, though semi-structured interviews are less prone to this bias than self-administered questionnaires. Nonetheless, when the symptoms of an Axis I disorder improve, the level of personality pathology usually decreases [13]. Thus, there is a false positive problem when assessing personality disorders in patients who are acutely symptomatic. As a result, some investigators evaluate personality disorders after resolution of Axis I symptomatology. On the other hand, a problem with the approach of delaying the assessment until symptom abatement is that it would result in the exclusion of patients who either never improved, or who relapsed and were symptomatic after an earlier period of improvement. Because Axis II pathology is associated with the chronicity of Axis I disorders [14,15], a study requiring improvement in Axis I symptom severity would disproportionately exclude patients with personality disorders, thereby artificially reducing the personality disorder prevalence rate. Studies of personality disorders in psychiatric patients need to balance the potential confounding influence of psychiatric state with the potential lack of generalizability of results based on patients who have improved in treatment.

How Should Personality Disorders be Diagnosed?

Clinical epidemiological studies, similar to other diagnostic research, should be based on structured research evaluations because structured research evaluations also improve diagnostic ascertainment when compared with unstructured diagnostic evaluations. Most of the research demonstrating problems with unstructured diagnostic evaluations has been done with Axis I disorders. One line of evidence suggesting diagnoses are under-recognized in clinical practice is a comparison of diagnostic comorbidity rates in studies using structured versus unstructured interviews. A review of this literature found much lower comorbidity rates in studies using unstructured clinical evaluations versus studies using structured research evaluations [16]. Some reports more directly suggest disorder under-detection. In a study by Davidson and Smith [17], a history of trauma was assessed in 54 outpatients immediately after they completed their unstructured clinical diagnostic evaluation. Seven (13%) patients were diagnosed with current posttraumatic stress disorder, only one of whom received the diagnosis from their intake clinician. Markowitz and colleagues [18] administered the Structured Clinical Interview for DSM-IV (SCID) to 90 outpatients and diagnosed 34 with dysthymic disorder. A review of 30 of the 34 dysthymic patients' clinical charts revealed that the diagnosis of dysthymic disorder was considered in the differential diagnosis by intake clinicians in less than half the cases.

Zimmerman and Mattia [16] examined whether diagnostic comorbidity is generally less frequently identified during a routine clinical evaluation than a semi-structured diagnostic interview. Axis I diagnoses derived from structured and unstructured clinical interviews were compared in two groups of psychiatric outpatients seen in the same practice setting. Of individuals presenting for an intake appointment to a general adult psychiatric practice, 500 underwent a routine unstructured clinical interview. Subsequent to the completion of the first study, the method of conducting diagnostic evaluations was changed and 500 individuals were interviewed with the SCID. The two groups had similar demographic characteristics and scored similarly on paper-and-pencil symptom questionnaires. Individuals interviewed with the SCID were assigned significantly more Axis I diagnoses than individuals who were assessed with an unstructured interview. More than one-third of patients interviewed with the SCID were diagnosed with three or more disorders, in contrast to fewer than 10% of the patients assessed with an unstructured interview. Fifteen disorders were more frequently diagnosed in the SCID sample, and these differences cut across mood, anxiety, eating, somatoform, and impulse control disorder categories. The results therefore suggested that in routine clinical practice, clinicians markedly under-recognized diagnostic comorbidity.

Shear and colleagues [19] questioned whether clinicians apply DSM-IV diagnostic criteria in a rigorous manner, and suggested that clinical diagnoses may not be very accurate. This hypothesis is consistent with the results of a nationwide survey done by Zimmerman and colleagues [20,21] several years earlier, which found that psychiatrists use the DSM primarily for reimbursement purposes and not because they believe that the diagnostic criteria are reliable or valid. Shear and colleagues [19] interviewed 164 psychiatric outpatients with the SCID after they were evaluated clinically. More diagnoses were made on the SCID. The two most noteworthy findings were that more than one-third of patients were diagnosed with adjustment disorder by the clinicians versus only 7% by the SCID interviewers, and that only 13% of the patients diagnosed by clinicians were given an anxiety disorder diagnosis, whereas more than half (53%) of the patients interviewed with the SCID were diagnosed with a current anxiety disorder. The investigators also found that half of the patients with a current primary diagnosis of major depressive disorder on the SCID were diagnosed with adjustment disorder by clinicians. Shear and colleagues concluded that clinicians' diagnoses are often inaccurate, and that this poses a barrier to the implementation of treatments that have proven effective for specific disorders.

In a study in Texas of 200 community mental health patients, Basco and colleagues [22] administered the SCID to the patients as a test of the utility of research diagnostic procedures in clinical practice. They found that supplementing information from the patients' charts with the information from the

SCID resulted in more than five times as many comorbid conditions being diagnosed (223 versus 41 comorbid diagnoses being made).

With regards to personality disorder recognition, Zimmerman and Mattia [23] examined the impact of assessment methodology on the prevalence rate of borderline personality disorder and found that the disorder was much less frequently diagnosed with an unstructured clinical evaluation than with a semi-structured diagnostic interview. The validity of the semi-structured diagnostic interview was suggested by the finding that when the information from the semi-structured interview was presented to the treating clinicians, borderline personality disorder was much more likely to be diagnosed. Further evidence of the validity of the semi-structured research interview diagnosis came from a comparison of the demographic and clinical characteristics of the patients with and without borderline personality disorder in which predicted differences were found [24].

A similar result was found in a study of patients with obsessive-compulsive disorder (OCD). Tenney and colleagues [25] evaluated 65 outpatients with OCD and found that 29% were diagnosed with a personality disorder on the basis of an unstructured clinical interview, lower than the 50.8% who were administered the SCID-II. Molinari and colleagues [26] compared rates of DSM-III-R personality disorders diagnosed according to the structured interview for DSM-III-R personality (SIDP-R) and an unstructured clinical interview in consecutively admitted patients to a gerosychiatric unit. Patients who were significantly cognitively impaired or actively psychotic were excluded. The final sample of 200 patients included 100 male patients hospitalized on a geropsychiatric unit of a Veterans Affairs (VA) medical center and 100 female patients hospitalized on a geropsychiatric unit at a private hospital. Separate interviewers were used in the two sites. Thus, this article can be considered to represent two independently conducted studies of personality disorder diagnoses in geropsychiatric inpatients. The data in Table 1 shows that in both sites significantly more patients were diagnosed with any personality disorder based on the SIDP-R. The prevalence rates of the specific disorders were generally low; however, for every disorder more diagnoses were made according to the SIDP-R than the unstructured clinical interview.

Thus, there is little debate that unstructured clinical interviews cannot be relied upon to form the basis of prevalence rates of personality disorders in clinical practice. It should be noted that there is a different type of debate in the field regarding the most valid method of assessing personality disorders. Specifically, the validity of semi-structured diagnostic interviews to assess personality disorders has been challenged because these interviews, which rely on direct questions to ascertain the presence or absence of the personality disorder criteria, differ from the methods clinicians use to diagnose personality disorders [27]. Clinicians, rather than relying on direct questioning at a single interview, typically use a longitudinal perspective to determine the presence or absence of a personality disorder, and their judgments are based on the real life vignettes patients describe during the course of treatment and the behavior and attitudes

Table 1
DSM-III-R personality disorder rates in two samples of geropsychiatric inpatients diagnosed by an unstructured clinical interview and the SIDP-R

	VA sample (n = 100)		Private hospital (n = 100)	
	Clinical	SIDP-R	Clinical	SIDP-R
Paranoid	1%	26%***	1%	8%*
Schizoid	1%	6%	0%	5%*
Schizotypal	0%	9%**	0%	2%
Antisocial	2%	4%	0%	2%
Borderline	2%	8%	1%	5%
Histrionic	0%	12%***	0%	7%**
Narcissistic	0%	5%*	0%	2%
Avoidant	0%	18%***	0%	5%*
Dependent	8%	9%	2%	9%*
Obsessive	2%	17%***	0%	7%**
Passive-aggressive	0%	12%***	0%	4%
PDNOS	11%	11%	0%	4%
Any PD	27%	61%***	4%	52%***

*$P < 0.05$.
**$P < 0.01$.
***$P < 0.001$.
Data from Molinari V, Ames A, Essa M. Prevalence of personality disorders in two geropsychiatric inpatient units. J Geriatr Psychiatry Neurol 1994;7:209–15.

patients display during the treatment sessions. Although there is some controversy as to how to best assess personality disorders, at the present time the semi-structured interview remains the most widely used method in research. Moreover, a large amount of literature examining the treatment, prognostic, familial, and biological correlates of personality disorders indicates that diagnosing personality disorders with a semi-structured interview is valid [28].

What Should be Included as a Personality Disorder?
The DSM-IV provides criteria for 10 personality disorders in the official text (schizoid, schizotypal, paranoid, antisocial, borderline, histrionic, narcissistic, avoidant, dependent, and obsessive-compulsive) as well as two disorders in the appendix requiring further study (depressive and negativistic). In addition, a residual not otherwise specified (NOS) disorder can be diagnosed in individuals with significant personality pathology that does not meet the criteria for any specific disorder. Exactly how frequent personality disorders are in psychiatric patients will therefore depend, in part, on which disorders are included in the investigation.

CLINICAL EPIDEMIOLOGICAL STUDIES OF PERSONALITY DISORDERS
Clinical epidemiological studies do not use the same sophisticated sampling methods that are used in community-based epidemiological studies. The authors

Table 2
Prevalence of DSM personality disorders in clinical epidemiological studies

Author	Patients	Criteria	Interview	Any PD	PARA	ZOID	TYPAL	ANTI	BORD	HIST	NARC	AVOID	DEPEN	OC
Dahl [47]	231 consecutively admitted inpatients, more than half of whom had a substance use disorder and no patient was diagnosed with major depression	DSM-III	SADS & SIB	44.6	0.5	2.7	22.0	18.2	20.3	19.3	1.6	9.1	2.1	0.5
Fabrega [51]	18,179 patients evaluated in a diagnostic evaluation center	DSM-III	Clinical	12.9	0.2	0.2		2.2	2.1		0.3			
Fossati [37]	431 consecutively admitted patients (213 inpatients, 218 outpatients), the most frequent Axis I diagnoses being anxiety and eating disorders	DSM-IV	SCID-II	71.9	6.3	1.2	4.6	4.6	22.5	13.7	35.7	5.1	3.0	5.1
Grilo [49]	117 consecutively admitted young adults (age 18–37)	DSM-IIIR	PDE	65.8	4.3	2.6	8.5	13.7	42.7	9.4	6.0	12.8	15.4	3.4
Herpertz [52]	231 consecutively admitted inpatients	DSM-III-R	AMPS	36.5	4.2	11.5	1.2	3.7	13.6	19.8	8.6	18.5	13.6	48.1
Kantojarvi [53]	444 hospitalized subjects	DSM-III-R	Clinical	14.6	0.1	0.0	0.1	4.5	5.6	0.1	0.1	0.1	0.1	0.0
Kass [31]	609 consecutively evaluated patients in residents outpatient clinic	DSM-III	Clinical	51.1	4.9	1.0	3.9	1.9	11.0	6.1	2.9	4.9	8.0	1.9

Study	Description	Criteria	Method											
Koenigsberg [32]	2,462 psychiatric patients from every level of care (inpatient, outpatient, emergency clinic, C-L service) evaluated by psychiatry residents	DSM-III	Clinical	35.9	0.4	0.0	1.9	1.9	12.3	2.8	0.9	1.0	2.8	0.8
Kunik [54]	547 consecutively evaluated inpatients aged 50 and over	DSM-III	Clinical	12.6										
Marinangeli [46]	156 consecutive inpatients, half of whom had a mood disorder	DSM-IIIR	SCID-II	73.7	27.6	5.1	6.4	10.3	40.4	13.5	25.6	28.2	20.5	34.6
Mezzich [55]	1,111 consecutive evaluated patients in a diagnostic evaluation center with a wide range of Axis I disorders, the most frequent being mood (30.7%) and substance use disorders (26.6%)	DSM-III	Clinical	21.9										
Molinari [26]	100 consecutively admitted male patients to a VA geropsychiatric inpatient unit, and 100 consecutively admitted female patients to a geropsychiatric unit of a private hospital. Psychotic and cognitively impaired patients excluded.	DSM-III-R	SIDP-R	56.5	17.0	5.5	5.5	3.0	6.5	9.5	3.5	11.5	9.0	12.0
			Clinical	14.5	1.0	0.5	0.0	1.0	1.5	0.0	0.0	0.0	5.0	1.0

(continued on next page)

Table 2
(continued)

Author	Patients	Criteria	Interview	Any PD	PARA	ZOID	TYPAL	ANTI	BORD	HIST	NARC	AVOID	DEPEN	OC
Oldham [33]	100 consecutive applicants for outpatient psychoanalysis, about one-third of whom had a mood or anxiety disorder	DSM-IIIR	PDE		4.0	1.0	0.0	4.0	18.0	5.0	6.0	16.0	6.0	10.0
Oldham [45]	129,286 in- and outpatients served by the New York state mental health facilities	DSM-III	Clinical	10.8										
Ottosson [48]	138 patients from a variety of settings	DSM-IV	DIP-I	65.9	21.0	4.3	8.0	10.1	33.3	5.8	5.1	37.0	9.4	28.3
Stangl [50]	119 inpatients and 12 outpatients with a variety of Axis I diagnoses	DSM-III	SIDP	51.1	0.8	0.8	9.1	3.8	22.1	22.9	3.8	11.4	13.0	5.3

Abbreviations: AMPS, Aachen list of items for the registration of personality disorders; ANTI, antisocial PD; AVOID, avoidant PD; BORD, borderline PD; C-L service, consultation and liaison; DEPEN, dependent PD; DIP, DSM-IV and ICD-10 personality questionnaire; HIST, histrionic PD; ICD-10, International Classification of Diseases; NARC, narcissistic PD; OC, obsessive-compulsive PD; PARA, paranoid PD; PD, personality disorder; PDE, personality disorders evaluation; PDNOS, personality disorder not otherwise specified; SADS, Schedule for Affective Disorders and Schizophrenia; SIB, Schedule for Interviewing Borderlines; TYPAL, schizotypal PD; ZOID, schizoid PD.

include in their review studies of consecutively ascertained samples, with minimal exclusion criteria that were not enriched with patients who had a personality disorder. Therefore, the authors did not include a large study of 1,760 patients interviewed with the structured interview for DSM-IV personality (SIDP-IV) who were referred for psychotherapy [29] for personality pathology because the rates in this sample would be artificially elevated. Likewise, the authors did not include the numerous studies of homogeneous samples of patients with a single, or limited number, or axis I disorders. These studies are often conducted in research centers that are of uncertain generalizability to community-based treatment facilities. The authors also did not included studies that excluded patients with common, nonpsychotic disorders. For example, Okasha and colleagues [30] evaluated personality disorders in neurotic outpatients with a diagnosis of an anxiety, somatoform, adjustment, or dissociative disorder. Because patients with mood disorders were excluded, the authors did not include this study.

The authors identified 16 clinical epidemiological studies of personality disorders. The methods and results of these studies are summarized in Table 2. All of the clinical epidemiological surveys of 500 patients or larger, except the one conducted in the authors clinical-research practice, have been based on unstructured clinical evaluations [31–33]. By far the largest study is Oldham and Skodol's study of more than 125,000 patients (approximately 60% outpatients) in the New York State mental health system. The 11% rate of any personality disorder in this study is similar to the rates reported in community-based epidemiological studies [34]. Oldham and Skodol, themselves, suggested that personality disorders were likely underdiagnosed by the clinicians in their study.

Including Oldham and Skodol's study, in seven of the studies diagnoses were based on unstructured clinical interviews, and in one study diagnoses based on unstructured and structured interviews were reported. The frequency of any personality disorder was less than 20% in five of these eight studies. In contrast, in seven of the eight studies using a semi-structured diagnostic interview, more than 40% of the patients were diagnosed with a personality disorder.

The Rhode Island Methods to Improve Diagnostic Assessment and Services (MIDAS) project is the largest clinical epidemiological study using semi-structured interviews assessing a wide range of psychiatric disorders conducted in a general clinical outpatient practice [35]. Among the strengths of the study are that diagnoses are based on the reliable and valid procedures used in research studies, and the patients are presenting to a community-based psychiatric outpatient practice rather than a research clinic specializing in the treatment of one or a few disorders.

The MIDAS project represents an integration of research methodology into a community-based outpatient practice affiliated with an academic medical center [35]. Patients have been recruited in the MIDAS project from the Rhode Island Hospital Department of Psychiatry outpatient practice. This private practice group predominantly treats individuals with medical insurance (including Medicare but not Medicaid) on a fee-for-service basis, and it is distinct from the hospital's outpatient residency training clinic that predominantly serves lower income, uninsured, and medical assistance patients.

A comprehensive diagnostic evaluation is conducted upon presentation for treatment. During the course of the MIDAS project, the assessment battery has changed. The assessment of all DSM-IV personality disorders was not introduced until the study was well underway and the procedural details of incorporating research interviews into the clinical practice had been well established. The authors administered the full SIDP-IV [36] to 859 patients. The data in Table 3 shows the demographic and diagnostic characteristics of the sample. The majority of the subjects were white, female, married or single, and had some college education. The mean age of the sample was 37.8 years (standard deviation = 11.9). The most frequent DSM-IV diagnoses were major depressive disorder (47.9%), social phobia (26.5%), generalized anxiety disorder (17.5%), and panic disorder (17.0%).

Slightly less than one-third of the subjects was diagnosed with one of the 10 DSM-IV personality disorders (31.4%, $n = 270$). When the subjects with personality disorder NOS are included, the rate of any personality disorder increased to almost half of the sample (45.5%, $n = 391$). Of the 270 subjects meeting criteria for one of the specific personality disorders, 60.4% ($n = 163$) had more than one personality disorder, and 25.2% ($n = 68$) had two or more personality disorders. The data in Table 4 indicate that the most frequent specific personality disorder was avoidant personality disorder (14.7%). Personality disorder NOS and avoidant personality disorder were the only personality disorders diagnosed in more than 10% of the subjects, and seven personality disorders were diagnosed in less than 5%. Histrionic and avoidant personality disorder were the most likely to be diagnosed as the sole personality disorder, whereas more than half the subjects diagnosed with each of the other personality disorders were diagnosed with another personality disorder.

The results from the MIDAS project, consistent with the results of other clinical epidemiological studies using semi-structured interviews, indicate that personality disorders are frequent in psychiatric outpatients. Exactly how frequent depends, in part, on the breadth of definition. When limited to the 10 DSM-IV personality disorders defined by specified criteria, approximately one-third of the patients were diagnosed with a personality disorder. The prevalence increased by about 15% to 45.5% when the residual personality disorder NOS category was included. The authors did not include the DSM-IV appendix diagnoses in the prevalence estimate, though other investigators have done so [37]. The authors examined the validity of depressive personality disorder and reported that its prevalence was 22%, which would have made it the most frequent personality disorder in the authors' patients [38]. The decision not to include the appendix diagnoses was made because they are not part of the official nomenclature. Their inclusion would have, of course, increased the overall prevalence of any personality disorder. Thus, the seemingly straightforward question of the prevalence rate of personality disorders is

Table 3
Demographic characteristics and current Axis I diagnoses of 859 psychiatric outpatients evaluated in the MIDAS project

Characteristic	n	%
Gender		
Female	527	61.4
Male	332	36.8
Education		
<12 years	83	9.7
High school graduate or GED	214	24.9
Some college	338	39.3
College graduate	224	26.1
Marital status		
Married	334	38.9
Living with someone	61	7.1
Widowed	12	1.4
Separated	55	6.4
Divorced	124	14.7
Never married	273	31.8
Race		
White	752	87.5
Black	32	3.7
Hispanic	22	2.6
Asian	10	1.2
Portuguese	32	3.7
Other	11	1.3
Age (years)	$M = 37.0$	$SD = 12.2$
Current DSM-IV diagnosis[a]		
Major depression	384	44.7
Bipolar I depression	16	1.9
Bipolar II depression	24	2.8
Dysthymic disorder	59	6.9
Generalized anxiety disorder	180	21
Panic disorder without agoraphobia	34	4
Panic disorder with agoraphobia	108	12.6
Social phobia	239	27.8
Specific phobia	97	11.3
Obsessive-compulsive disorder	61	7.1
Posttraumatic stress disorder	92	10.7
Adjustment disorder	50	5.8
Schizophrenia	4	0.5
Schizoaffective disorder	4	0.5
Bulimia nervosa	10	1.2
Binge eating disorder	25	2.9
Alcohol abuse/dependence	85	9.9
Drug abuse/dependence	46	5.4
Somatization disorder	4	0.5
Undifferentiated somatoform disorder	26	3
Hypochondriasis	13	1.5

[a]Individuals could be given more than one diagnosis.

Table 4
Frequency of DSM-IV personality disorders in 859 psychiatric outpatients evaluated with the SIDP-IV

	Total n (%)	n (%) without another PD
Paranoid	36 (4.2)	6 (16.7)
Schizoid	12 (1.4)	2 (16.7)
Schizotypal	5 (0.6)	1 (20)
Antisocial	31 (3.6)	13 (41.9)
Borderline	80 (9.3)	26 (32.5)
Histrionic	9 (1)	6 (66.7)
Narcissistic	20 (2.3)	4 (20)
Avoidant	126 (14.7)	74 (58.7)
Dependent	12 (1.4)	4 (33.3)
Obsessive-compulsive	75 (8.7)	37 (49.3)
Not otherwise specified	121 (14.1)	121 (100)
Cluster A	48 (5.6)	
Cluster B	112 (13)	
Cluster C	187 (21.8)	
Any personality disorder	391 (45.5)	

complicated by the decision of how wide a net to cast in defining a personality disorder.

As described earlier, other methodological issues that can influence personality disorder prevalence rates include the timing of the assessment, the presence of Axis I disorders, the source of information, and the instrument used [13]. The authors conducted the assessment when patients presented for treatment, and thus were symptomatic with an Axis I disorder.

Another reason for conducting Axis II assessments during the initial evaluation is that this is when treatment decisions are usually made. A thorough personality disorder assessment at the time of the initial evaluation aids case formulation and decisions about treatment approaches. Finally, despite the possible bias from state effects, assessments made when patients are symptomatic have strong, consistent, prognostic value [9].

Another methodological issue that can affect prevalence rates is the source of the information. Several studies have found poor levels of agreement between patients and informants in diagnosing personality disorders [39–42]. Adding information from an informant interview to the information already ascertained from patients nearly doubles the prevalence of personality disorders [43]. However, the validity of personality disorder diagnoses based on patient information alone was as high as that based on information from both patients and informants [44]. The authors are not aware of any study suggesting that information from informants increases the validity of personality disorder diagnoses based on patient information alone; thus, assessment was limited to the patients.

Personality disorder prevalence rates are affected by the type of diagnostic interview conducted. More diagnoses are made according to semi-structured interviews rather than unstructured clinical evaluations. The three studies that compared prevalence rates as a function of assessment methodology in patients ascertained from the same setting clearly demonstrated that more diagnoses were made by the semi-structured interview [23,25,26].

A final factor that can influence personality disorder prevalence rates is the demographic and clinical profile of the patients evaluated. Questions of generalizability can be raised about the MIDAS project, as with every other clinical epidemiology study. In contrast to community-based epidemiological studies that use sophisticated sampling methods to ensure representation of the general population, clinical epidemiological studies are generally single site studies of samples of convenience. Patients who are applicants for psychoanalysis [45] or long-term inpatient treatment of personality disorders [45] are likely to have higher rates of personality disorders than unselected patient series.

Variability in methods, samples, and diagnostic criteria makes it difficult to assimilate the results of the present study with other clinical epidemiological studies of patients with a mixture of Axis I disorders. Most studies are of inpatients only [46,47], or inpatients combined with outpatients [31,32,37,45,48–50]. The authors are not aware of a study that is comparable to the MIDAS project in which semi-structured interviews have been integrated into a community-based outpatient practice. Clinical epidemiological studies using semi-structured interviews tend to be done on inpatient settings because the patients are a captive audience. Integrating research quality evaluations into an outpatient practice requires that more obstacles are overcome [35]. Diagnostic interviewers in the studies listed in Table 2 have included psychiatric residents [31,32,46], trained research interviewers with undescribed levels of experience and professional training [37,49], and psychiatrists with extensive prior experience with semi-structured diagnostic interviews [48]. The samples also differ in the most frequent Axis I disorders and the diagnostic system used. Despite these differences, some conclusions can be drawn from these studies. Studies using standardized interviews consistently diagnose almost half or more of patients with a personality disorder. Thus, the frequency of personality disorders is high, and clinicians need to be vigilant to their presence because of the potential impact on treatment planning and prognosis. Borderline personality disorder was one of the two most frequent diagnoses in almost every study, whereas schizoid personality disorder was infrequently diagnosed in almost all studies. This is consistent with the general pattern of cluster B diagnoses being the most frequent, and cluster A diagnoses the least frequent disorders.

Personality disorder NOS, operationally defined as falling within one criterion of the DSM-IV threshold on two or more specific personality disorders, was the most frequent diagnosis in the authors' sample. Perhaps interviews such as the SIDP-IV, which are thematically organized around content areas rather than by diagnosis, increase the probability of subthreshold diagnoses. Interviews such as the SIDP-IV were intended to be less prone to halo effects in which ratings of individual criteria are influenced by how close the individual is to meeting the criteria for the disorder. Most clinical epidemiological studies of outpatients did not include the personality disorder NOS category, though in two other studies, one using a thematically organized interview [49] and the other using an unstructured clinical evaluation [32], personality disorder NOS was one of the most common diagnoses. From a nosological perspective, the relatively high frequency of subthreshold diagnoses lends support to the dimensional rather than categorical approach toward classification.

In conclusion, personality disorders are frequent in psychiatric settings. A summary of clinical epidemiological studies using semi-structured diagnostic interviews indicates that approximately half of patients have a personality disorder, thus making these disorders, as a group, among the most frequent disorders treated by psychiatrists. Personality disorders should be evaluated in every patient because their presence can influence the course and treatment of the Axis I disorder, which patients typically identify as their chief complaint.

References

[1] Olfson M, Marcus SC, Druss B, et al. National trends in the outpatient treatment of depression. JAMA 2002;287:203–9.

[2] Kessler RC, Zhao S, Katz SJ, et al. Past-year use of outpatient services for psychiatric problems in the National Comorbidity Survey. Am J Psychiatry 1999;156:115–23.

[3] Narrow WE, Regier DA, Rae DS, et al. Use of services by persons with mental and addictive disorders: findings from the National Institute of Mental Health Epidemiologic Catchment Area Program. Arch Gen Psychiatry 1993;50:95–107.

[4] Goodwin R, Hoven C, Lyons J, et al. Mental health service utilization in the United States. The role of personality factors. Soc Psychiatry Psychiatr Epidemiol 2002;37: 561–6.

[5] Alegria M, Bijl R, Lin E, et al. Income differences in persons seeking outpatient treatment for mental disorders: a comparison of the United States with Ontario and the Netherlands. Arch Gen Psychiatry 2000;57:383–91.

[6] Berkson J. Limitations of the application of fourfold table analysis to hospital data. Biometric Bulletin 1946;2:47–53.

[7] Farmer R, Nelson-Gray R. Personality disorders and depression: hypothetical relations, empirical findings, and methodological considerations. Clin Psychol Rev 1990;10:453–76.

[8] Alnaes R, Torgersen S. Personality and personality disorders predict development and relapses of major depression. Acta Psychiatr Scand 1997;95:336–42.

[9] McDermut W, Zimmerman M. The effects of personality disorders on outcome in the treatment of depression. In: Rush AJ, editor. Mood and anxiety disorders. Philadelphia: Williams & Wilkins; 1998. p. 321–38.

[10] Shea M, Widiger T, Klein M. Comorbidity of personality disorders and depression: Implications for treatment. J Consult Clin Psychol 1992;60:857–68.

[11] Yeomans F, Clarkin J, Kernberg O. A primer of transference focused psychotherapy for the borderline patient. New Jersey: Jason Aronson; 2002.

[12] Zimmerman M, Pfohl B, Stangl D, et al. Assessment of DSM-III personality disorders: the importance of interviewing an informant. J Clin Psychiatry 1986;47:261–3.

[13] Zimmerman M. Diagnosing personality disorders: a review of issues and research methods. Arch Gen Psychiatry 1994;51:225–45.

[14] Reich JH, Green AI. Effect of personality disorders on outcome of treatment. J Nerv Ment Dis 1991;179:74–82.

[15] Rothschild L, Zimmerman M. Interface between personality and depression. In: Fava M, Alpert J, editors. Handbook of chronic depression. New York: Marcel Dekker; 2004. p. 19–48.

[16] Zimmerman M, Mattia JI. Psychiatric diagnosis in clinical practice: Is comorbidity being missed? Compr Psychiatry 1999;40:182–91.
[17] Davidson J, Smith R. Traumatic experiences in psychiatric outpatients. J Trauma Stress 1993;3:459–75.
[18] Markowitz JC, Moran ME, Kocsis JH, et al. Prevalence and comordibity of dysthymic disorder among psychiatric outpatients. J Affect Disord 1991;24:63–71.
[19] Shear MK, Greeno C, Kang J, et al. Diagnosis of nonpsychotic patients in community clinics. Am.J. Psychiatry 2000;157:581–7.
[20] Zimmerman M, Jampala V, Sierles F, et al. DSM-IV: a nosology sold before its time? Am J Psychiatry 1991;148:463–7.
[21] Zimmerman M, Jampala VC, Sierles FS, et al. DSM-III and DSM-IIIR: What are American psychiatrists using and why? Compr Psychiatry 1993;181:360–4.
[22] Basco MR, Bostic JQ, Davies D, et al. Methods to improve diagnostic accuracy in a community mental health setting. Am J Psychiatry 2000;157:1599–605.
[23] Zimmerman M, Mattia JI. Differences between clinical and research practice in diagnosing borderline personality disorder. Am J Psychiatry 1999;156:1570–4.
[24] Zimmerman M, Mattia JI. Axis I diagnostic comorbidity and borderline personality disorder. Compr Psychiatry 1999;40:245–52.
[25] Tenney NH, Schotte CK, Denys DA, et al. Assessment of DSM-IV personality disorders in obsessive-compulsive disorder: comparison of clinical diagnosis, self-report questionnaire, and semi-structured interview. J Personal Disord 2003;17:550–61.
[26] Molinari V, Ames A, Essa M. Prevalence of personality disorders in two geropsychiatric inpatient units. J Geriatr Psychiatry Neurol 1994;7:209–15.
[27] Westen D. Divergences between clinical and research methods for assessing personality disorders: Implications for research and the evolution of Axis II. Am J Psychiatry 1997;154:895–903.
[28] Livesley W. Handbook of personality disorders. Theory, research and treatment. New York: The Guilford Press; 2001.
[29] Verheul R, Bartak A, Widiger T. Prevalence and construct validity of personality disorder not otherwise specified (PDNOS). J Personal Disord 2007;21:359–70.
[30] Okasha A, Omar AM, Lotaief F, et al. Comorbidity of Axis I and Axis II diagnoses in a sample of Egyptian patients with neurotic disorders. Compr Psychiatry 1996;37:95–101.
[31] Kass F, Skoldol AE, Charles E, et al. Scaled ratings of DSM-III personality disorders. Am J Psychiatry 1985;142:627–30.
[32] Koenigsberg HW, Kaplan RD, Gilmore MM, et al. The relationship between syndrome and personality disorder in DSM-III: experience with 2,462 patients. Am J Psychiatry 1985;142:207–12.
[33] Oldham JM, Skodol AE. Personality disorders in the public sector. Hosp Community Psychiatry 1991;42:481–7.
[34] Mattia J, Zimmerman M. Epidemiology of personality disorders. In: Livesley J, editor. Handbook of personality disorders. New York: Guilford Press; 2001. p. 107–23.
[35] Zimmerman M. Integrating the assessment methods of researchers in routine clinical practice: the Rhode Island Methods to Improve Diagnostic Assessment and Services (MIDAS) project. In: First M, editor, Standardized evaluation in clinical practice, vol. 22. Washington, DC: American Psychiatric Publishing, Inc. 2003. p. 29–74.
[36] Pfohl B, Blum N, Zimmerman M. Structured interview for DSM-IV personality. Washington, DC: American Psychiatric Press, Inc.; 1997.
[37] Fossati A, Maffei C, Bagnato M, et al. Patterns of covariation of DSM-IV personality disorders in a mixed psychiatric sample. Compr Psychiatry 2000;41:206–15.
[38] McDermut W, Zimmerman M, Chelminski I. The construct validity of depressive personality disorder. J Abnorm Psychol 2003;112:49–60.
[39] Modestin J, Puhan A. Comparison of assessment of personality disorder by patients and informants. Psychopathology 2000;33:265–70.

[40] Molinari V, Kunik M, Mulsant B, et al. The relationship between patient, informant, social worker, and consensus diagnoses of personality disorders in elderly depressed patients. Am J Geriatr Psychiatry 1998;6:136–44.

[41] Bernstein D, Kasapis C, Bergman A, et al. Assessing Axis II disorders by informant interview. J Personal Disord 1997;11:158–67.

[42] Riso L, Klein D, Anderson R, et al. Concordance between patients and informants on the personality disorder examination. Am J Psychiatry 1994;151:568–73.

[43] Zimmerman M, Pfohl B, Coryell W, et al. Diagnosing personality disorder in depressed patients. A comparison of patient and informant interviews. Arch Gen Psychiatry 1988;45:733–7.

[44] Zimmerman M, Pfohl B, Coryell W, et al. Personality disorder diagnoses: who should we interview?, in 143rd Annual Meeting of the Psychiatric Association. New York, 1990.

[45] Oldham JM, Skodol AE, Kellman HD, et al. Comorbidity of Axis I and Axis II disorders. Am J Psychiatry 1995;152:571–8.

[46] Marinangeli M, Butti G, Scinto A, et al. Patterns of comorbidity among DSM-III-R personality disorders. Psychopathology 2000;33:69–74.

[47] Dahl AA. Some aspects of DSM-III personality disorders illustrated by a consecutive sample of hospitalized patients. Acta Psychiatr Scand 1986;73:61–7.

[48] Ottosson H, Bodlund O, Ekselius L, et al. DSM-IV and ICD-10 personality disorders: a comparison of a self-report questionnaire (DIP-Q) with a structured interview. Eur Psychiatry 1998;13:246–53.

[49] Grilo C, McGlashan T, Quinlan D, et al. Frequency of personality disorders in two age cohorts of psychiatric inpatients. Am J Psychiatry 1998;155:140–2.

[50] Stangl D, Pfohl G, Zimmerman M, et al. A structured interview for the DSM-III personality disorders. Arch Gen Psychiatry 1985;42:591–6.

[51] Fabrega H Jr, Ulrich R, Pilkonis P, et al. Personality disorders diagnosed at intake at a public psychiatric facility. Hosp Community Psychiatry 1993;44:159–62.

[52] Herpertz S, Steinmeyer EM, Sass H. "Patterns of comorbidity" among DSM-III-R and ICD-10 personality disorders as observed with a new inventory for the assessment of personality disorders. Eur Arch Psychiatry Clin Neurosci 1994;244:161–9.

[53] Kantojarvi L, Veijola J, Laksy K, et al. Comparison of hospital-treated personality disorders and personality disorders in a general population sample. Nord J Psychiatry 2004;58:357–62.

[54] Kunik ME, Mulsant BH, Rifai AH, et al. Diagnostic rate of comorbid personality disorder in elderly psychiatric inpatients. Am J Psychiatry 1994;151:603–5.

[55] Mezzich J, Coffman G, Goodpastor S. A format for DSM-III diagnostic formulation: experience with 1,111 consecutive patients. Am J Psychiatry 1982;139:591–6.

Genetics of Personality Disorders

Ted Reichborn-Kjennerud, MD[a,b,c],*

[a]Division of Mental Health, Department of Adult Mental Health, Norwegian Institute of Public Health, Box 4404 Nydalen, N-0403 Oslo, Norway
[b]Institute of Psychiatry, University of Oslo, P.O. Box 1130 Blindern, 0318 Oslo, Norway
[c]Department of Epidemiology, Columbia University, 722 West 168th Street, New York, NY 10032, USA

This review of the literature on genetic contributions to the etiology of personality disorders broadly follows the *Diagnostic and Statistical Manual of Mental Disorders* (DSM) classification. Until recently, relatively few genetic studies of personality disorders as defined by this system had been published [1]. I therefore begin by evaluating the current evidence for genetic influences on the DSM axis II disorders. The field of psychiatric genetics has for a long time been moving beyond simple quantitative genetic studies [2]. Advanced quantitative methods are now being applied to explore the nature and mode of action of genetic risk factors. In the field of personality disorder, researchers are beginning to address issues like whether genetic risk factors are specific to a given personality disorder, or also influence the liability to other personality disorders or axis I disorders, and to what extent genetic influences are stable over time or change as a function of the developmental stage of the individual. One of the most exciting directions in psychiatric genetics is the rapidly developing field of molecular genetic studies aiming to identify specific genes correlated with psychiatric phenotypes. Personality disorders, like most other psychiatric diagnostic categories, are etiologically complex, which implies that they are influenced by several genes and several environmental factors. The interplay between genes and the environment is a field that is receiving increasing attention and is addressed both in relation to quantitative and molecular methods. Finally, future directions are discussed.

THE PHENOTYPES

The current DSM-IV classification [3] includes 10 categorical personality disorder diagnoses grouped into three clusters (A, B, and C) and two personality disorders listed in Appendix B. The second-order cluster classification gives the system a hierarchical structure, which implies that genetic influence can in part

*Division of Mental Health, Department of Adult Mental Health, Norwegian Institute of Public Health, Box 4404 Nydalen, N-0403 Oslo, Norway. *E-mail address*: ted.reichborn kjennerud@fhi.no

0193-953X/08/$ – see front matter
doi:10.1016/j.psc.2008.03.012

be specific to each personality disorder or trait and in part general to all disorders or traits in a cluster (see later in this article). It is also possible that personality disorders share genetic risk factors in common with disorders in other clusters.

The most controversial and long-standing issue in the field is whether personality disorders should be conceptualized dimensionally or as discrete categories. There seems to be a general agreement that personality disorders are best classified dimensionally [4–6]. Many alternative systems are, however, discussed for DSM-V (see Krueger and colleagues [7]). Recent studies have, for example, provided empirical support for the validity of a system based on dimensional representations of the current DSM-IV categories [8,9].

The understanding of the role of genetic factors in the etiology of disorders and traits is inseparably linked to classification, since a precise definition of the phenotype is a prerequisite for all successful genetic studies. The DSM classification system serves many purposes and is mainly based on phenotypic similarities and not designed specifically for genetic studies. This is a problem not only in the genetics of personality disorders, and the search for better phenotypes for genetic studies is especially well illustrated in the literature on schizophrenia (eg, Gottesman and Gould [10], Fanous and Kendler [11], and Braff and colleagues [12]).

QUANTITATIVE GENETIC STUDIES
Methods
The basic goals of family, twin, and adoption studies are to quantify the degree to which individual liability to a disorder results from familial effects (in family studies) or genetic factors (in twin and adoption studies). These methods are therefore often referred to as *quantitative genetics* in contrast to *molecular genetics* [13].

Twin studies have been most commonly used to estimate the specific effects of genetic risk factors on personality disorders. This is usually called heritability and is defined as the proportion of phenotypic differences between individuals (or proportion of variance) in a particular population that can be attributed to genetic differences. Genetic effects can be additive, meaning that the independent effects of different alleles or loci act in an additive way to increase risk for the disorder or trait, or nonadditive, which means that different alleles interact (epistasis or dominance). In classical twin studies the environmental effects are divided into common or shared environment, which includes all environmental exposures that contribute to making twins similar, and individual-specific or unique environment, which includes all environmental exposures that make twins different, plus measurement error. The total variance in a phenotype is partitioned into three variance components, each accounted for by three latent variables: additive genetic, shared environment, and individual-specific environment. This means that the genetic and environmental effects are not measured, ie, we do not know which genes or which environmental factors influence the phenotype.

The statistical model upon which modern twin studies are based is called the liability-threshold model [14], and assumes that a large number of genetic and environmental risk factors with small individual effects are involved, resulting in a distribution of liability or risk in the population that approximates normality. A dichotomous disorder will appear when a certain threshold is exceeded. An alternative model assumes that disorders in themselves are actually also phenotypically continuous, ie, that a disorder exists on a continuum from normal to abnormal [13]. Twin studies can be used regardless of whether personality disorders are defined categorically or dimensionally, but the statistical power of the classical twin study with categorically defined phenotypes is much lower than if the phenotype is ordinal or continuous [15].

If heritability has been established, several more complex models can be employed to explore the nature and mode of action of the genetic risk factors [2]. Multivariate analyses [16] can, for example, be used to explore to what extent genetic and environmental risk factors are specific to a given personality disorder or shared in common with other personality disorders or axis I disorders, and if genetic effects differ over time in a developmental perspective.

In the traditional models of disease etiology in psychiatric epidemiology, the causal pathway is conceptualized as moving from the environment to the organism. However, since genes influence behavior, genetic factors can indirectly influence or control exposure to the environment [16,17], often called *gene-environment correlation* [13].

Genetic factors can also control an individual's sensitivity to the environment, ie, genetic factors can alter an organism's response to environmental stressors [16–18]. This is usually called *gene-environment interaction* [18]. In quantitative studies, genetic factors are not measured, but are either inferred (eg, disorder in biological parent in adoption studies) or modeled as a latent variable in twin studies [17,19].

Empirical Studies
Normal and abnormal personality traits
Normal personality traits have been repeatedly shown to be influenced by genetic factors with heritability estimates ranging from approximately 30% to 60% [20,21]. The genetic effects are mainly additive, but nonadditive contributions of a smaller magnitude have been identified in studies with sufficient statistical power. Shared environmental factors are usually found to be of minor or no importance [20]. Similar heritability estimates have been found in studies using a dimensional classification system for personality disorders based on self-report [22,23].

Numerous studies have shown that DSM personality disorders can be represented by models of normal personality (eg, Trull [24]). On the phenotypic level, relatively high correlations have been found, for example, between higher order factors of the five-factor model and DSM personality disorders [25,26]. No behavior genetic study of the relationship between normal personality and personality disorders as defined by the DSM system has, however, been published.

DSM personality disorders
Most of the early quantitative genetic studies of DSM or DSM-like personality disorders investigated antisocial and schizotypal personality disorder using

a variety of measures. The first twin study based on structured interviews that included all DSM personality disorders was published by Torgersen and colleagues [27] in 2000. It was based on DSM-III and DSM-III-R diagnoses, and used data from a mixed clinical sample where at least one of the twins had been treated for a major mental disorder. Standard errors were not presented but the small sample size suggests that they would have been substantial. The method of ascertainment also suggests that results from this study should be interpreted with caution. More recent studies have used data from a large population-based twin sample recruited from the Norwegian Institute of Public Health Twin Panel that was assessed with structured interviews for both DSM-IV axis I and axis II disorders (referred to as the "Axis I–Axis II Twin Study" later in this article). Instead of categorical diagnoses, dimensional representations of the personality disorders based on the number of criteria endorsed were used in the analyses of this sample (eg, Kendler and colleagues [28] and Reichborn-Kjennerud and colleagues [29]).

Cluster A disorders. Prior studies have suggested that familial/genetic factors contribute to the etiology of the three personality disorders making up DSM Cluster A: paranoid, schizoid, and schizotypal personality disorder [30]. A series of twin studies that examined various measures of schizoid, schizotypal, and paranoid-like traits using self-report questionnaires have been published (eg, Kendler and colleagues [31], Claridge and Hewitt [32], Kendler and Hewitt [33], Linney and colleagues [34], and Jang and colleagues [35]). These studies have nearly uniformly found significant genetic influences on these traits and failed to find shared environmental effects. Heritabilities are typically most frequently in the range of 35% to 60%. In a twin study based on a clinical sample, Torgersen and colleagues [27] found lower heritability estimates for paranoid personality disorder (28%) and schizoid personality disorder (29%), but much high heritability for schizotypal personality disorder (61%). In a more recent multivariate study of DSM-IV cluster A personality disorders using data from the Axis I–Axis II Twin Study, Kendler and colleagues [28] estimated heritability to be 21% for paranoid, 28% for schizotypal, and 26% for schizoid personality disorder. No shared environmental effects or sex differences were found. The proportion of genetic liability that was shared in common with the other cluster A disorders were 100% for schizotypal personality disorder, 43% for paranoid personality disorder, and 29% for schizoid personality disorder, suggesting that schizotypal personality disorder had the strongest genetic relationship to the common genetic liability to the cluster A disorders.

In twin studies, unreliability of measurement will decrease the heritability estimates. Although the inter-rater reliability in the Kendler and colleagues above-mentioned study was excellent, the test-retest reliability or stability of measurement for personality disorders has been shown to be imperfect [36]. It is also possible that genetic and environmental risk factors assessed by self-report questionnaires versus interviews are different. A second study from the same sample was therefore undertaken [37]. Data from a self-report questionnaire study conducted in 1998 were used in addition to the above-mentioned interview data to account for unreliability of measurement by using two measures differing in both time and mode of assessment. The results indicated that the liability to cluster A personality disorders was substantially higher than in the first study, with estimated heritabilities of 66% for paranoid personality disorder, 55% to 59% for schizoid personality disorder, and 72% for schizotypal personality disorder.

Cluster B disorders. Antisocial personality disorder is by far the most studied personality disorder in cluster B using genetic epidemiological methods. In a meta-analyses of 51 twin and adoption studies on antisocial behavior based largely on records, self-report, and family-report, Rhee and Waldman [38] found that the variance could most parsimoniously be explained by additive genetic factors (32%), nonadditive genetic factors (9%), shared environmental factors (16%), and individual-specific environmental factors (43%). There were no significant differences in the magnitude of genetic and environmental influences for males and females. In a twin study based on a clinical sample, heritability estimates for the other three cluster B personality disorders were found to be 69% for borderline, 63% for histrionic, and 77% for narcissistic personality disorder [27]. More recently, Torgersen and colleagues [39] conducted a population-based twin study of dimensional representations of the cluster B personality disorders based on data from the Axis I–Axis II Twin Study. Heritability was estimated to be 38% for antisocial personality disorder, 31% for histrionic personality disorder, 24% for narcissistic personality disorder, and 35% for borderline personality disorder. No shared environmental influences or sex or effects were found. The most parsimonious multivariate model included one genetic factor influencing all four cluster B personality disorders, and one genetic factor influencing only antisocial personality disorder and borderline personality disorder, in addition to specific genetic factors for each personality disorder. Antisocial personality disorder had the highest and borderline and histrionic personality disorder had the lowest disorder-specific genetic variance. These results suggest that borderline and histrionic personality disorder best represent the overall genetic liability to cluster B. Borderline personality disorder and antisocial personality disorder appear to share genetic and environmental risk factors above and beyond that due to the genetic and environmental factors common to all four cluster B personality disorders, indicating that, etiologically, cluster B has a "substructure" in which antisocial personality disorder and borderline personality disorder are more closely related to each other than to the other cluster B disorders.

Cluster C disorders. The so called "Anxious" cluster includes avoidant, dependent, and obsessive-compulsive personality disorder. In a clinically ascertained twin study, heritability estimates for avoidant, dependent, and obsessive-compulsive personality disorder were found to be 28%, 57%, and 77%, respectively [27]. In a multivariate study of DSM-IV cluster C personality disorders, based on data from the Axis I–Axis II Twin Study [29], heritability estimates were found to be 35% for avoidant personality disorder, 31% for dependent personality disorder, and 27% for obsessive-compulsive personality disorder. No shared environmental effects or sex differences were found. A genetic factor common to all cluster C personality disorders accounted for 83% of the genetic influence in avoidant personality disorder, 48% in dependent personality disorder, and 15% in obsessive-compulsive personality disorder, indicating that avoidant personality disorder had the strongest genetic relationship to the common genetic liability to the cluster C disorders. Common genetic and environmental factors accounted for only 11% of the variance in obsessive-compulsive personality disorder, indicating that obsessive-compulsive personality disorder is mostly etiologically distinct from the two other cluster C personality disorders.

Disorders in appendix B. In a population-based twin study of depressive personality disorder, using data from the Axis I–Axis II Twin Study, Ørstavik and colleagues [40] found that liability could best be explained by additive genetic and unique environmental factors alone, with heritability estimates of 49% in females and 25% in males. Unlike the results for the other DSM-IV personality disorders, both quantitative and qualitative sex differences were found corresponding to findings from studies on major depression [41].

Data from the Axis I–Axis II Twin Study were also used to examine DSM-IV passive-aggressive personality disorder [42]. Significant familial aggregation was found. The prevalence of endorsed passive-aggressive personality disorder criteria in this community sample was, however, too low to conclude with confidence regarding the relative influence of genetic and shared environmental factors.

Personality disorders and axis I disorders
Several lines of evidence indicate specific axis I/axis II relationships [43,44], and the underlying validity of the DSM axis I–axis II division has been questioned by a number of authors (eg, Siever and Davis [45], Widiger [46], and Krueger [47]). Behavior genetic studies can be used to evaluate the extent to which common genetic risk factors can account for the observed associations between personality disorders and axis I disorders.

Schizophrenia. A number of family and adoption studies have examined the risk for paranoid, schizoid, and schizotypal personality disorder in relatives of schizophrenic and control probands. While a few studies can be found where all three cluster A personality disorders are at increased risk in relatives of schizophrenic probands [48,49], more common are studies that find that only schizotypal personality disorder [50–54] or schizotypal personality disorder and paranoid personality disorder [55] have a significant familial relationship with schizophrenia. These results suggest that schizotypal personality disorder is the personality disorder with the closest familial relationship to schizophrenia, followed by paranoid personality disorder and then schizoid personality disorder. This order—schizotypal, paranoid, and schizoid personality disorder—is the same as for the proportion of genetic risk due to the common genetic factor observed in the multivariate study of cluster A personality disorders mentioned earlier [28]. The congruence of these results is consistent with the hypothesis that the common genetic risk factor for cluster A personality disorders reflects, in the general population, the liability to schizophrenia. The extended phenotype believed to reflect this genetic vulnerability is often described by the term schizophrenia-spectrum. Schizotypal personality disorder has been suggested to be the prototypical disorder in this spectrum [56]. In a recent family study, Fogelson and colleagues [57] showed that avoidant personality disorder, currently classified in DSM cluster C, also occurred more frequently in relatives of probands with schizophrenia even after controlling for schizotypal and paranoid personality disorder. This replicates findings from earlier studies [49,52], and suggest that avoidant personality disorder should also be included in this spectrum.

Substance use disorders. Numerous family, adoption, and twin studies have demonstrated that antisocial personality disorder, conduct disorders, and substance use disorders (often called externalizing disorders) share a common genetic liability (eg, Krueger and colleagues [58] and Kendler and colleagues [59]). In a recent, elegantly designed, family-twin study, Hicks and colleagues [60] found that a highly heritable (80%) general vulnerability to all the externalizing disorders accounted for most of the familial resemblance. Disorder-specific vulnerabilities were detected for conduct disorder, alcohol dependence, and drug dependence, but not for antisocial personality disorder. The same group has also reported an association between externalizing disorders and reduced amplitude of the P3 component of the brain event-related potential, suggesting that this could be a common biological marker of the biological vulnerability to these disorders [61].

Major depression. In a recent longitudinal population-based twin study, based on a very large sample, Kendler and colleagues [62] found that the personality trait neuroticism strongly predicted the risk for major depression, and that the association between the two disorders could be explained largely by shared genetic risk factors The genetic correlation between neuroticism and major depression was 0.46 for women and 0.47 for men.

Previous studies have found that depressive personality and mood disorders aggregate in families (eg, McDermut and colleagues [63]). In a bivariate twin study, Ørstavik and colleagues [64] used data from the Axis I–Axis II Twin Study to determine the sources of co-occurrence between depressive personality disorder and major depressive disorder. The results suggested that a substantial part of the covariation between the two disorders was accounted for by genetic factors. The genetic correlation between the two disorders was 0.56. Unlike in the study by Kendler and colleagues [62], no sex differences were found, but this could be due to lack of statistical power because of much smaller sample size. Family studies also indicate that borderline personality disorder and major depression share familial risk factors [65]. Preliminary results from analyses of data from the Axis I–Axis II Twin Study indicate that this can be attributed to common genetic liability, with a genetic correlation similar to that found for depressive personality disorder and major depression (Reichborn-Kjennerud and colleagues, unpublished data, December 2007).

Anxiety disorders. One of the most studied and controversial Axis I and Axis II relationships is that between social phobia and avoidant personality disorder. Using data from the Axis I–Axis II Twin Study, Reichborn-Kjennerud and colleagues [66] sought to determine the sources of co-occurrence between social phobia and dimensional representations of avoidant personality disorder by estimating to what extent the two disorders are influenced by common genetic and environmental factors. Only female-female pairs were included in this investigation. The model-fitting results indicated that avoidant personality disorder and social phobia share all their genetic risk factors and that the environmental risk factors for the two disorders were uncorrelated. Within the limits of statistical power, this suggests that, in females, there is a common genetic vulnerability to avoidant personality disorder and social phobia. An individual with high genetic liability will develop avoidant personality disorder versus social phobia entirely as a result of environmental risk factors unique to each disorder. The results from another recent study are in accordance with these findings. Using a similar method, Bienvenu and colleagues [67] found that genetic factors for neuroticism and extraversion accounted for all the genetic influence on DSM-IV social phobia and agoraphobia. The environmental correlations between the personality measures and the anxiety disorders were very low.

Gene-environment interplay
Gene-environment correlation. Twin and adoption studies have provided much of the evidence for gene-environment correlations by demonstrating genetic influences for a number of measures of the environment (for a review see Kendler and Baker [68]). Overall, the evidence from twin and adoption studies suggests that gene-environment correlations are mediated by heritable personality traits and possibly personality disorders [18,68,69]. Saudino and colleagues [70] demonstrated that all the genetic influence on controllable positive and negative life events could be explained by genetic factors influencing individual differences in personality traits such as neuroticism, extraversion, and openness to experience. Kendler and colleagues [71] showed that neuroticism was associated with an elevated risk for marital problems, job loss, financial difficulties, and problems getting along with people in their social network. It has also been shown that 30% to 42% of divorce heritability could be attributed to genetic factors affecting individual differences in personality in one of the spouses [72], and that the propensity to marry and marital satisfaction to a large extent could be accounted for by genetic factors influencing personality [73,74].

Gene-environment interaction. The initial indications that gene-environment interaction was likely to be operating came from adoption and twin studies (for a review see Tsuang and colleagues [75]). Gene-environment interaction was demonstrated in an adoption study as early as in 1974, when Crowe [76] found that early institutional care was a risk factor for later antisocial behavior only when a genetic risk factor was present. In another adoption study, Cadoret and colleagues [77] found significant gene-environment interaction by showing that there was a negligible risk for antisocial behavior from a genetic risk alone (antisocial behavior in the biological parent), no effect of an adverse adoptive family environment alone, but a substantial effect when both were present. In a later study with a similar design but with a larger number of adoptees, the finding was replicated [78]. Jaffe and colleagues [79], using a twin design, found significant gene-environment interaction with respect to childhood maltreatment and the development of antisocial behavior, and, in a twin study, Tuvblad and colleagues [80] demonstrated a significant gene-environment interaction by showing that the heritability for adolescent antisocial behavior is higher in socioeconomic advantaged environments. Using an advanced family design, Feinberg and colleagues [81] recently found an interaction of genotype and both parental negativity and low warmth predicting antisocial behavior. Significant gene-environment interaction has also been demonstrated in schizophrenia spectrum disorders. In an adoption study, Tienari and colleagues [82] showed that there was a significant association between disordered rearing and the diagnosis of schizophrenia spectrum disorder in the offspring of mothers with but not in offspring of mothers without the diagnoses.

Longitudinal studies. Most of the genetic studies that have investigated changes in genetic influences over time have used measures related to antisocial personality disorder. The following examples illustrate the potential of longitudinal quantitative genetic methods. In a twin study, Lyons and colleagues [83] demonstrated that the genetic influence on symptoms of DSM-III-R antisocial personality disorder was much more prominent in adulthood than in adolescence. Silberg and colleagues [84], studying twins between 10 and 17 years of age, found a single genetic factor that influenced antisocial behavior beginning at age 10 through young adulthood, a shared environmental effect beginning in adolescence, a transient genetic effect at puberty, and genetic influences specific to adult antisocial behavior. In another recent twin study of externalizing disorders, biometric analyses revealed increasing genetic variation and heritability for men but a trend toward decreasing genetic variation and increasing environmental effects for women [85].

MOLECULAR GENETIC STUDIES
Methods
The aims of molecular genetics are to determine the genomic location and identity of genes associated with a disorder, and to identify critical DNA variants and trace the biological pathways from DNA via gene product (protein) to disorder (see Kendler [2]). In this article we will deal only with the first of these.

If a disorder is defined categorically, the associated genetic variants are often called susceptibility genes; if the phenotype is defined dimensionally, the associated genetic variants are called quantitative trait loci (QTL) indicating multiple genetic variants that contribute to quantitative variation. As discussed earlier, personality disorders can be conceptualized either as categorical entities or as quantitative traits. Using a quantitative measure confers several advantages for molecular studies including increase in statistical power. It also makes possible to use an extreme selection design, enriched for trait-linked genetic variation, substantially reducing the amount of genotyping required for the detection of small-effect QTLs [86].

Traditionally, linkage and association studies have been most commonly used for mapping disease loci. Space limitations do not permit us to discuss these methods in detail here. They have been extensively reviewed elsewhere (eg, Sham and McGuffin [87]). The two methods have complementary properties in that linkage is only able to detect genes of major effects (eg, relative risk > 2 or 10% of the variance), whereas association studies can detect genes of minor effects (eg, relative risk < 2 or < 1% of the variance) [87]. The etiology of most common diseases is determined by multiple, relatively common, genetic variants and environmental factors, each of which have small effects and are neither necessary nor sufficient to individually cause the disease [88]. Recent research suggests that the effects of single genes for complex disorders are small (odds ratio [OR] < 1.5) [89]. Case-control association studies have therefore become the most popular design used in the search for common polymorphisms thought to underlie common complex traits or disorders [88]. They can be either *hypothesis-driven candidate gene studies* focusing on a particular gene or genome region, or *genome-wide association (GWA) analyses conducted without a prior hypothesis* [88]. GWA studies are based on the knowledge that the differences that are responsible for the heritability of complex disorders often involve a substitution of a single base pair, called single nucleotide polymorphisms (SNPs). An international database of common human sequence variation now includes over 3.1 million SNPs, which provides high coverage of common variants of the human genome [90].

The number of molecular genetic studies is increasing exponentially [91]; however, only a very small fraction of these are replicated [92,93]. Several explanations have been invoked, including publication bias, misclassification of outcome, phenotypic heterogeneity, allelic heterogeneity, weak prior probabilities of association, multiple testing, population stratification, and inadequate sample sizes and failure to take into account gene-gene and gene-environment interactions. Recently, criteria for replicating genotype-phenotype associations have been proposed to limit the "plethora of false-positive results" [94].

One of the strategies that have been suggested to increase the rate of success for molecular genetics in psychiatry is the use of so-called endophenotypes. An endophenotype is defined as a heritable characteristic that is along the pathway between a disorder and genotype and influences the disorder [10]. Because endophenotypes are presumed to be more proximal to the action of the genes and are more common than the disorder, it has been assumed that they can potentially have great value for psychiatric genetics. Personality traits have been suggested as endophenotypes for Axis I disorders; eg, schizotypy for schizophrenia [12], and neuroticism for major depression and generalized anxiety disorder [95]. It has also been suggested that an endophenotypic approach should be applied to personality disorders by using clinical dimensions such as affective instability, impulsivity, and aggression [96]. One of the main reasons for using endophenotypes is the belief that the effect sizes of loci contributing to endophenotypes are larger than those contributing to disorder susceptibility.

The number of genes involved in common diseases is not known, and depends on the gene frequency in the population [97]. The effect of a single gene may be contingent on the simultaneous presence of another gene or genes. New methods for dealing with interaction between genes have been developed (see Marchini and colleagues [98]) and an increasing number of gene-gene interaction studies are being published.

Gene-environment interaction using molecular methods provides more secure results than quantitative genetic studies by using identified susceptibility genes rather than unmeasured latent genetic factors [18]. Moffitt and colleagues [99] recently outlined strategies for studying interactions between measured genes and measured environments.

Empirical Studies

An enormous number of studies on the genetics of personality traits have been published during the past decade. A review of this literature is beyond the scope of this article. In the following, I will give a few examples of studies related to DSM personality disorders. Until further replications are published, these results must be considered tentative. Most of the studies are hypothesis-driven candidate gene association studies focusing on genes involved in the neurotransmitter pathways, especially in the serotonergic and dopaminergic systems. No GWA studies of personality disorders have yet been published.

Cluster A

Rosmond and colleagues [100] found that Cluster A personality disorders were associated with a polymorphism in the gene coding for the dopamine 2 receptor (DRD2). Using findings from quantitative genetic studies indicating that common genetic risk factors exist for shizotypal personality disorder and schizophrenia, Stefanis and colleagues [101] examined the potential impact of SNPs within the four most prominent candidate genes for schizophrenia. Dysbindin (DTNBP1) and D-amino-acid oxidase (DAAO) both showed associations with symptoms of schizotypy. Similarly, Fanous and colleagues [102], using a linkage approach, found that a subset of schizophrenia susceptibility genes also affect schizotypy in nonpsychotic relatives. Significant associations with schizotypal personality traits have also been found in several studies with polymorphisms in the gene coding for Catechol-O-methyltransferase (COMT), an enzyme involved in the degradation of catecholamines [103–105].

Cluster B

Polymorphisms in the gene coding for the enzyme monoamine oxidase A (MAOA), involved in the degradation of biogenic amines like serotonin and norepinephrin, have been found to be associated with cluster B personality disorders, but not with cluster C personality disorders [106]. Ni and colleagues [107] later found that the MAOA gene polymorphism was significantly associated with borderline personality disorder. The same group has also reported associations between borderline personality disorder and polymorphisms in the gene coding for the serotonin 5-HT2A receptor [108], and borderline personality disorder and polymorphisms in the serotonin transporter gene (5-HTTLPR) [109]. A main effect of the 5-HTTLPR polymorphism on borderline personality disorder in bulimic women was also reported by Steiger and colleagues [110]. Joyce and colleagues [111] found a significant association between borderline personality disorder and a polymorphism in the gene coding for the dopamine receptor DAT1 in depressed patients, and a polymorphism in the tryptophan hydroxylase-2 gene (TPH2T) has been linked to personality traits related to emotional instability as well as to cluster B and cluster C personality disorders [112].

Cluster C

Patients diagnosed with cluster C personality disorders have been found to have a significantly higher frequency of the short-form allele of the 5-HTTLPR [113]. It has previously been suggested that this polymorphism was associated with anxiety-related traits [114] but later studies have yielded conflicting results (see Munafo and colleagues [115]). Joyce [116] found an association between avoidant and obsessive compulsive personality disorder symptoms and the dopamine D3 receptor (DRD3) polymorphism. In a later study and a meta-analysis, the finding for obsessive compulsive symptoms were replicated leading the authors to conclude that DRD3 may contribute to the development of obsessive compulsive personality disorder [117].

Gene-environment correlation

Only recently, studies of gene-environment correlation using measured genes and measured environments have been published. Dick and colleagues [118] found that individuals who had a polymorphism in a gene (GABRA2) associated with alcohol dependence were less likely to be married, in part because they were at higher risk for antisocial personality disorder and were less likely to be motivated by a desire to please others. Homozygosity for an allele of the dopamine D2 receptor gene (DRD2) has been found to be associated with significantly more paternal rejection, and parental and paternal overprotection compared with individuals who were heterozygous [119].

Gene-environment interaction

Based on results from quantitative genetic studies showing gene-environment interaction for antisocial behavior, Caspi and colleagues [120] studied the association between childhood maltreatment and a functional polymorphism in the promoter region of the monoamine oxidase A (MAOA) gene on antisocial behavior assessed through a range of categorical and dimensional measures using questionnaire and interview data plus official records. The results showed no main effect of the gene, a main effect for maltreatment, and a substantial and significant interaction between the gene and adversity. The maltreated children whose genotype conferred low levels of MAOA expression more often developed conduct disorder and antisocial personality than children with a high-activity MAOA genotype. Foley and colleagues [121] replicated this finding and extended the initial analysis by showing that the gene-environment interaction could not be accounted for by gene-environment correlation. Other studies have failed to replicate the gene-environment interaction effect (eg, Huizinga and colleagues [122]). In a recent meta-analysis, however, the original finding was replicated. In addition, the findings were extended to include childhood (closer in time to the maltreatment), and the possibility of a spurious finding was ruled out by accounting for gene-environment correlation [123]. The interaction between MAOA and childhood maltreatment in the etiology of antisocial personality disorder appears to be one of the few replicated findings in the molecular genetics of personality disorders.

SUMMARY

All the DSM personality disorders appear to be modestly to moderately heritable, influenced in part by genetic factors common to all the personality disorders in the same cluster and in part by disorder specific influences. Varying degrees of overlapping genetic risk factors with specific axis I disorders has been found for some of the axis II disorders. Genotype-environment interplay has been demonstrated in numerous studies, and a few longitudinal studies have shown different influences of genetic factors at different developmental stages.

Despite the current focus on molecular genetic methods, quantitative genetic studies still have a role to play in the genetics of personality disorders. One of the many issues that needs to be addressed is the higher-order structure of the genetic risk factors underlying the liability to personality disorders. So far, no multivariate study of all 10 DSM personality disorders has been undertaken. Two main genetic factors have been shown to influence the most common axis I disorders [59], and multivariate studies including several axis I and axis II disorders could provide new important insights into the etiology of psychiatric disorders. Overlap in genetic liability could also be of potential interest to psychiatric nosology. However, the fundamental question is to what extent genotypic versus phenotypic similarities should guide psychiatric classification [124,125]. As pointed out by Kendler [125], genetic studies alone cannot address these nosologic issues and other potential validators have to be taken into consideration.

Molecular genetic studies of personality disorders as well as of normal personality and most other psychiatric phenotypes have so far been inconclusive. However, this field is moving very rapidly. Common patterns of genetic variation are now the basis for lower cost and more efficient genomics technologies, and comprehensive GWA studies in very large samples are being applied to several psychiatric phenotypes.

As illustrated above, one of the most urgent problems that has to be resolved before we can expect a breakthrough in this field is related to classification and selection of suitable phenotypes for genetic studies. It is highly unlikely that the new DSM-V classification of personality disorders will provide a solution. Although Flint and Munafo [86] in a recent meta-analysis of endophenotypic studies in psychiatry found that the effect sizes of the loci examined to date were no larger than for other phenotypes, the use of endophenotypes for personality disorders seems to be the most promising strategy [10,96].

References

[1] McGuffin P, Moffitt T, Thapar A. Personality disorders. In: McGuffin P, Owen MJ, Gottesman II, editors. Psychiatric genetics & genomics. Oxford (England): Oxford University Press; 2002. p. 183–210.

[2] Kendler KS. Psychiatric genetics: a methodologic critique. Am J Psychiatry 2005;162(1): 3–11.

[3] American Psychiatric Association. Diagnostic and statistical manual of mental disorders. 4th edition. Washington, DC: American Psychiatric Association; 1994.

[4] Oldham JM, Skodol AE. Charting the future of axis II. J Personal Disord 2000;14(1): 17–29.

[5] Widiger TA, Samuel DB. Diagnostic categories or dimensions? A question for the diagnostic and statistical manual of mental disorders—fifth edition. J Abnorm Psychol 2005;114(4):494–504.

[6] Widiger TA, Trull TJ. Plate tectonics in the classification of personality disorder—shifting to a dimensional model. Am Psychol 2007;62(2):71–83.

[7] Krueger RF, Skodol AE, Livesley WJ, et al. Synthesizing dimensional and categorical approaches to personality disorders: refining the research agenda for DSM-V Axis II. Int J Methods Psychiatr Res 2007;16:S65–73.

[8] Skodol AE, Oldham JM, Bender DS, et al. Dimensional representations of DSM-IV personality disorders: relationships to functional impairment. Am J Psychiatry 2005;162(10): 1919–25.

[9] Morey LC, Hopwood CJ, Gunderson JG, et al. Comparison of alternative models for personality disorders. Psychol Med 2007;37(7):983–94.

[10] Gottesman II, Gould TD. The endophenotype concept in psychiatry: etymology and strategic intentions. Am J Psychiatry 2003;160(4):636–45.

[11] Fanous AH, Kendler KS. Genetic heterogeneity, modifier genes, and quantitative phenotypes in psychiatric illness: searching for a framework. Mol Psychiatry 2005;10(1):6–13.

[12] Braff DL, Freedman R, Schork NJ, et al. Deconstructing schizophrenia: an overview of the use of endophenotypes in order to understand a complex disorder. Schizophr Bull 2007;33(1):21–32.

[13] Plomin R, DeFries JC, McClearn GE, et al. Behavior genetics. New York: Worth Publishers; 2001.

[14] Falconer DS. The inheritance of liability to certain diseases, estimated from the incidence among relatives. Ann Hum Genet 1965;29:51–76.

[15] Neale MC, Eaves LJ, Kendler KS. The power of the classical twin study to resolve variation in threshold traits. Behav Genet 1994;24(3):239–58.

[16] Kendler KS. Twin studies of psychiatric illness: an update. Arch Gen Psychiatry 2001;58(11):1005–14.

[17] Kendler KS, Prescott CA. Genes, environment, and psychopathology. New York: The Guilford Press; 2006.

[18] Rutter M, Moffitt TE, Caspi A. Gene-environment interplay and psychopathology: multiple varieties but real effects. J Child Psychol Psychiatry 2006;47(3–4):226–61.

[19] Purcell S, Sham P. Variance components models for gene-environment interaction in quantitative trait locus linkage analysis. Twin Res 2002;5(6):572–6.

[20] Bouchard TJ, Loehlin JC. Genes, evolution, and personality. Behav Genet 2001;31(3): 243–73.

[21] Ando J, Suzuki A, Yamagata S, et al. Genetic and environmental structure of Cloninger's temperament and character dimensions. J Personal Disord 2004;18(4):379–93.

[22] Jang KL, Livesley WJ, Vernon PA, et al. Heritability of personality disorder traits: a twin study. Acta Psychiatr Scand 1996;94(6):438–44.

[23] Livesley WJ, Jang KL, Vernon PA. Phenotypic and genetic structure of traits delineating personality disorder. Arch Gen Psychiatry 1998;55(10):941–8.

[24] Trull TJ. Dimensional models of personality disorder: coverage and cutoffs. J Personal Disord 2005;19(3):262–82.

[25] Dyce JA, O'Connor BP. Personality disorders and the five-factor model: a test of facet-level predictions. J Personal Disord 1998;12(1):31–45.

[26] Morey LC, Gunderson JG, Quigley BD, et al. The representation of borderline, avoidant, obsessive-compulsive, and schizotypal personality disorders by the five-factor model. J Personal Disord 2002;16(3):215–34.

[27] Torgersen S, Lygren S, Oien PA, et al. A twin study of personality disorders. Compr Psychiatry 2000;41(6):416–25.

[28] Kendler KS, Czajkowski N, Tambs K, et al. Dimensional representations of DSM-IV Cluster A personality disorders in a population-based sample of Norwegian twins: a multivariate study. Psychol Med 2006;36(11):1583–91.

[29] Reichborn-Kjennerud T, Czajkowski N, Neale MC, et al. Genetic and environmental influences on dimensional representations of DSM-IV cluster C personality disorders: a population-based multivariate twin study. Psychol Med 2007;37(5):645–53.

[30] Parnas J, Licht D, Bovet P. Cluster A personality disorders: a review. In: Maj M, Akiskal H, Mezzich JE, editors. Personality disorders. Chichester (England): John Wiley & Sons Ltd; 2005. p. 1–74.

[31] Kendler KS, Heath A, Martin NG. A genetic epidemiologic study of self-report suspiciousness. Compr Psychiatry 1987;28(3):187–96.

[32] Claridge G, Hewitt JK. A biometrical study of schizotypy in a normal population. Pers Individ Dif 1987;8:303–12.

[33] Kendler KS, Hewitt JK. The structure of self-report schizotypy in twins. J Personal Disord 1992;6:1–17.

[34] Linney YM, Murray RM, Peters ER, et al. A quantitative genetic analysis of schizotypal personality traits. Psychol Med 2003;33(5):803–16.

[35] Jang KL, Woodward TS, Lang D, et al. The genetic and environmental basis of the relationship between schizotypy and personality—a twin study. J Nerv Ment Dis 2005;193(3):153–9.

[36] McGlashan TH, Grilo CM, Sanislow CA, et al. Two-year prevalence and stability of individual DSM-IV criteria for schizotypal, borderline, avoidant, and obsessive-compulsive personality disorders: toward a hybrid model of axis II disorders. Am J Psychiatry 2005;162(5):883–9.

[37] Kendler KS, Myers J, Torgersen S, et al. The heritability of cluster A personality disorders assessed by both personal interview and questionnaire. Psychol Med 2007;37(5):655–65.

[38] Rhee SH, Waldman ID. Genetic and environmental influences on antisocial behavior: a meta-analysis of twin and adoption studies. Psychol Bull 2002;128(3):490–529.

[39] Torgersen S, Czajkowski N, Jacobson K, et al. Dimensional representations of DSM-IV cluster B personality disorders in a population-based sample of Norwegian twins: a multivariate study. Psychol Med 2008 Feb 14;1–9 [E-pub ahead of print].

[40] Ørstavik RE, Kendler KS, Czajkowski N, et al. Genetic and environmental contributions to depressive personality disorder in a population-based sample of Norwegian Twins. J Affect Disord 2007;99(1–3):181–9.

[41] Kendler KS, Gatz M, Gardner CO, et al. A Swedish national twin study of lifetime major depression. Am J Psychiatry 2006;163(1):109–14.

[42] Czajkowski N, Kendler KS, Jacobson KC, et al. Passive-aggressive (negativistic) personality disorder: a population-based twin study. J Personal Disord 2008;22(1): 109–22.

[43] Tyrer P, Gunderson J, Lyons M, et al. Extent of comorbidity between mental state and personality disorders. J Personal Disord 1997;11(3):242–59.

[44] Dolan-Sewell RT, Krueger RF, Shea MT. Co-occurrence with syndrome disorders. In: Livesley WJ, editor. Handbook of personality disorders: theory, research and treatment. New York: The Guilford Press; 2001. p. 84–104.

[45] Siever LJ, Davis KL. A psychobiological perspective on the personality disorders. Am J Psychiatry 1991;148(12):1647–58.

[46] Widiger TA. Personality disorder and axis I psychopathology: the problematic boundary of axis I and axis II. J Personal Disord 2003;17(2):90–108.

[47] Krueger RF. Continuity of axes I and II: toward a unified model of personality, personality disorders, and clinical disorders. J Personal Disord 2005;19(3):233–61.

[48] Parnas J, Cannon TD, Jacobsen B, et al. Lifetime DSM-III-R diagnostic outcomes in the offspring of schizophrenic mothers. Results from the Copenhagen high-risk study. Arch Gen Psychiatry 1993;50(9):707–14.

[49] Kendler KS, McGuire M, Gruenberg AM, et al. The Roscommon family study. III. Schizophrenia-related personality disorders in relatives. Arch Gen Psychiatry 1993;50(10):781–8.

[50] Kety SS, Wender PH, Jacobsen B, et al. Mental illness in the biological and adoptive relatives of schizophrenic adoptees. Replication of the Copenhagen study in the rest of Denmark. Arch Gen Psychiatry 1994;51(6):442–55.

[51] Onstad S, Skre I, Edvardsen J, et al. Mental disorders in first-degree relatives of schizophrenics. Acta Psychiatr Scand 1991;83(6):463–7.

[52] Asarnow RF, Nuechterlein KH, Fogelson D, et al. Schizophrenia and schizophrenia-spectrum personality disorders in the first-degree relatives of children with schizophrenia: the UCLA family study. Arch Gen Psychiatry 2001;58(6):581–8.

[53] Tienari P, Wynne LC, Laksy K, et al. Genetic boundaries of the schizophrenia spectrum: evidence from the Finnish adoptive family study of schizophrenia. Am J Psychiatry 2003;160(9):1587–94.

[54] Torgersen S, Onstad S, Skre I, et al. Schizotypal personality disorder: a study of co-twins and relatives of schizophrenic probands. Am J Psychiatry 1993;150(11):1661–7.

[55] Baron M, Gruen R, Rainer JD, et al. A family study of schizophrenic and normal control probands: implications for the spectrum concept of schizophrenia. Am J Psychiatry 1985;142(4):447–55.

[56] Siever L, Davis KL. The pathopysiology of schizophrenia disorders: perspectives from the spectrum. Am J Psychiatry 2004;161:398–413.

[57] Fogelson DL, Nuechterlein KH, Asarnow RA, et al. Avoidant personality disorder is a separable schizophrenia-spectrum personality disorder even when controlling for the presence of paranoid and schizotypal personality disorders—The UCLA family study. Schizophr Res 2007;91(1–3):192–9.

[58] Krueger RF, Hicks BM, Patrick CJ, et al. Etiologic connections among substance dependence, antisocial behavior, and personality: modeling the externalizing spectrum. J Abnorm Psychol 2002;111(3):411–24.

[59] Kendler KS, Prescott CA, Myers J, et al. The structure of genetic and environmental risk factors for common psychiatric and substance use disorders in men and women. Arch Gen Psychiatry 2003;60(9):929–37.

[60] Hicks BM, Krueger RF, Iacono WG, et al. Family transmission and heritability of externalizing disorders—a twin-family study. Arch Gen Psychiatry 2004;61(9): 922–8.

[61] Hicks BM, Bernat E, Malone SM, et al. Genes mediate the association between P3 amplitude and externalizing disorders. Psychophysiology 2007;44(1):98–105.

[62] Kendler KS, Gatz M, Gardner CO, et al. Personality and major depression—a Swedish longitudinal, population-based twin study. Arch Gen Psychiatry 2006;63(10):1113–20.

[63] McDermut W, Zimmerman M, Chelminski I. The construct validity of depressive personality disorder. J Abnorm Psychol 2003;112(1):49–60.

[64] Ørstavik RE, Kendler KS, Czajkowski N, et al. The relationship between depressive personality disorder and major depressive disorder: a population-based twin study. Am J Psychiatry 2007;164:1866–72.

[65] Riso LP, Klein DN, Anderson RL, et al. A family study of outpatients with borderline personality disorder and no history of mood disorder. J Personal Disord 2000;14(3):208–17.

[66] Reichborn-Kjennerud T, Czajkowski N, Torgersen S, et al. The relationship between avoidant persinality disorder and social phobia: a population-based twin study. Am J Psychiatry 2007;164:1722–8.

[67] Bienvenu OJ, Hettema JM, Neale MC, et al. Low extraversion and high neuroticism as indices of genetic and environmental risk for social phobia, agoraphobia, and animal phobia. Am J Psychiatry 2007;164:1714–21.

[68] Kendler KS, Baker JH. Genetic influences on measures of the environment: a systematic review. Psychol Med 2007;37(5):615–26.

[69] Jaffee SR, Price TS. Gene-environment correlations: a review of the evidence and implications for prevention of mental illness. Mol Psychiatry 2007;12(5):432–42.

[70] Saudino KJ, Pedersen NL, Lichtenstein P, et al. Can personality explain genetic influences on life events? J Pers Soc Psychol 1997;72(1):196–206.

[71] Kendler KS, Gardner CO, Prescott CA. Personality and the experience of environmental adversity. Psychol Med 2003;33(7):1193–202.

[72] Jockin V, Mcgue M, Lykken DT. Personality and divorce: a genetic analysis. J Pers Soc Psychol 1996;71(2):288–99.

[73] Johnson W, Mcgue M, Krueger RF, et al. Marriage and personality: a genetic analysis. J Pers Soc Psychol 2004;86(2):285–94.

[74] Spotts EL, Lichtenstein P, Pedersen N, et al. Personality and marital satisfaction: a behavioural genetic analysis. European Journal of Personality 2005;19(3):205–27.

[75] Tsuang MT, Bar JL, Stone WS, et al. Gene-environment interactions in mental disorders. World Psychiatry 2004;3:73–83.

[76] Crowe RR. An adoption study of antisocial personality. Arch Gen Psychiatry 1974;31: 785–91.

[77] Cadoret RJ, Cain CA, Crowe RR. Evidence for gene-environment interaction in the development of adolescent antisocial behavior. Behav Genet 1983;13:301–10.

[78] Cadoret RJ, Yates WR, Troughton E, et al. Genetic-environmental interaction in the genesis of aggressivity and conduct disorders. Arch Gen Psychiatry 1995;52(11):916–24.

[79] Jaffee SR, Caspi A, Moffitt TE, et al. Nature X nurture: genetic vulnerabilities interact with physical maltreatment to promote conduct problems. Dev Psychopathol 2005;17(1):67–84.

[80] Tuvblad C, Grann M, Lichtenstein P. Heritability for adolescent antisocial behavior differs with socioeconomic status: gene-environment interaction. J Child Psychol Psychiatry 2006;47(7):734–43.

[81] Feinberg ME, Button TMM, Neiderhiser JM, et al. Parenting and adolescent antisocial behavior and depression—evidence of genotype x parenting environment interaction. Arch Gen Psychiatry 2007;64(4):457–65.

[82] Tienari P, Wynne LC, Sorri A, et al. Genotype-environment interaction in schizophrenia-spectrum disorder—long-term follow-up study of Finnish adoptees. Br J Psychiatry 2004;184:216–22.

[83] Lyons MJ, True WR, Eisen SA, et al. Differential heritability of adult and juvenile antisocial traits. Arch Gen Psychiatry 1995;52(11):906–15.

[84] Silberg JL, Rutter M, Tracy K, et al. Etiological heterogeneity in the development of antisocial behavior: the Virginia twin study of adolescent behavioral development and the young adult follow-up. Psychol Med 2007;37(8):1193–202.

[85] Hicks BM, Blonigen DM, Kramer MD, et al. Gender differences and developmental change in externalizing disorders from late adolescence to early adulthood: a longitudinal twin study. J Abnorm Psychol 2007;116(3):433–47.

[86] Flint J, Munafo MR. The endophenotype concept in psychiatric genetics. Psychol Med 2007;37(2):163–80.

[87] Sham P, McGuffin P. Linkage and association. In: McGuffin P, Owen MJ, Gottesman II, editors. Psychiatric genetics & genomics. Oxford, England: Oxford University Press; 2002. p. 55–73.

[88] Zondervan KT, Cardon LR. Designing candidate gene and genome-wide case-control association studies. Nat Protoc 2007;2:2492–501.

[89] Ioannidis JPA, Trikalinos TA, Khoury MJ. Implications of small effect sizes of individual genetic variants on the design and interpretation of genetic association studies of complex diseases. Am J Epidemiol 2006;164(7):609–14.

[90] The international HapMap Consortium 2. A second generation human haplotype map of over 3.1 million SNPs. Nature 2007;449:851–62.

[91] Munafo MR, Flint J. Meta-analysis of genetic association studies. Trends Genet 2004;20(9):439–44.

[92] Ioannidis JPA, Ntzani EE, Trikalinos TA, et al. Replication validity of genetic association studies. Nat Genet 2001;29(3):306–9.

[93] Hirschhorn JN, Lohmueller K, Byrne E, et al. A comprehensive review of genetic association studies. Genet Med 2002;4(2):45–61.

[94] NCI-NHGRI Working Group on Replication in Association Studies. Replicating genotype-phenotype associations. Nature 2007;447:655–60.

[95] Kuo PH, Neale MC, Riley BP, et al. A genome-wide linkage analysis for the personality trait neuroticism in the Irish affected sib-pair study of alcohol dependence. Am J Med Genet B Neuropsychiatr Genet 2007;144(4):463–8.

[96] Siever LJ. Endophenotypes in the personality disorders. Dialogues Clin Neurosci 2005;7: 139–51.

[97] Yang QH, Khoury MJ, Friedman JM, et al. How many genes underlie the occurrence of common complex diseases in the population? Int J Epidemiol 2005;34(5): 1129–37.

[98] Marchini J, Donnelly P, Cardon LR. Genome-wide strategies for detecting multiple loci that influence complex diseases. Nat Genet 2005;37:413–7.

[99] Moffitt TE, Caspi A, Rutter M. Strategy for investigating interactions between measured genes and measured environments. Arch Gen Psychiatry 2005;62(5):473–81.

[100] Rosmond R, Rankinen T, Chagnon M, et al. Polymorphism in exon 6 of the dopamine D-2 receptor gene (DRD2) is associated with elevated blood pressure and personality disorders in men. J Hum Hypertens 2001;15(8):553–8.

[101] Stefanis NC, Trikalinos TA, Avramopoulos D, et al. Impact of schizophrenia candidate genes on schizotypy and cognitive endophenotypes at the population level. Biol Psychiatry 2007;62(7):784–92.

[102] Fanous AH, Neale MC, Gardner CO, et al. Significant correlation in linkage signals from genome-wide scans of schizophrenia and schizotypy. Mol Psychiatry 2007;12(10): 958–65.

[103] Avramopoulos D, Stefanis NC, Hantoumi I, et al. Higher scores of self reported schizotypy in healthy young males carrying the COMT high activity allele. Mol Psychiatry 2002;7(7): 706–11.

[104] Stefanis NC, van Os J, Avramopoulos D, et al. Variation in catechol-O-methyltransferase val(158) met genotype associated with schizotypy but not cognition: a population study in 543 young men. Biol Psychiatry 2004;56(7):510–5.

[105] Schurhoff F, Szoke A, Chevalier F, et al. Schizotypal dimensions: an intermediate phenotype associated with the COMT high activity allele. Am J Med Genet B Neuropsychiatr Genet 2007;144(1):64–8.

[106] Jacob CP, Muller J, Schmidt M, et al. Cluster B personality disorders are associated with allelic variation of monoamine oxidase A activity. Neuropsychopharmacology 2005;30(9):1711–8.

[107] Ni XQ, Sicard T, Bulgin N, et al. Monoamine oxidase A gene is associated with borderline personality disorder. Psychiatr Genet 2007;17(3):153–7.

[108] Ni XQ, Bismil R, Chan K, et al. Serotonin 2A receptor gene is associated with personality traits, but not to disorder, in patients with borderline personality disorder. Neurosci Lett 2006;408(3):214–9.

[109] Ni XQ, Chan K, Bulgin N, et al. Association between serotonin transporter gene and borderline personality disorder. J Psychiatr Res 2006;40(5):448–53.

[110] Steiger H, Richardson J, Joober R, et al. The 5HTTLPR polymorphism, prior maltreatment and dramatic-erratic personality manifestations in women with bulimic syndromes. J Psychiatry Neurosci 2007;32(5):354–62.

[111] Joyce PR, Mchugh PC, McKenzie JM, et al. A dopamine transporter polymorphism is a risk factor for borderline personality disorder in depressed patients. Psychol Med 2006;36(6): 807–13.

[112] Gutknecht L, Jacob C, Strobel A, et al. Tryptophan hydroxylase-2 gene variation influences personality traits and disorders related to emotional dysregulation. Int J Neuropsychopharmacol 2007;10(3):309–20.

[113] Jacob CP, Strobel A, Hohenberger K, et al. Association between allelic variation of serotonin transporter function and neuroticism in anxious cluster C personality disorders. Am J Psychiatry 2004;161(3):569–72.

[114] Lesch KP, Bengel D, Heils A, et al. Association of anxiety-related traits with a polymorphism in the serotonin transporter gene regulatory region. Science 1996;274(5292): 1527–31.

[115] Munafo MR, Clark T, Flint J. Does measurement instrument moderate the association between the serotonin transporter gene and anxiety-related personality traits? A meta-analysis. Mol Psychiatry 2005;10(4):415–9.

[116] Joyce PR, Rogers GR, Miller AL, et al. Polymorphisms of DRD4 and DRD3 and risk of avoidant and obsessive personality traits and disorders. Psychiatry Res 2003;119(1–2):1–10.

[117] Light KJ, Joyce PR, Luty SE, et al. Preliminary evidence for an association between a dopamine D3 receptor gene variant and obsessive-compulsive personality disorder in patients with major depression. Am J Med Genet B Neuropsychiatr Genet 2006;141(4):409–13.

[118] Dick DM, Agrawal A, Shuckit MA, et al. Marital status, alcohol dependence, and GRBRA2: evidence for gene-environment correlation and interaction. J Stud Alcohol 2006;67:185–94.

[119] Lucht M, Barnow S, Schroeder W, et al. Negative perceived paternal parenting is associated with dopamine D-2 receptor exon 8 and GABA(A) alpha 6 receptor variants: An explorative study. Am J Med Genet B Neuropsychiatr Genet 2006;141(2):167–72.

[120] Caspi A, McClay J, Moffitt TE, et al. Role of genotype in the cycle of violence in maltreated children. Science 2002;297(5582):851–4.

[121] Foley DL, Eaves LJ, Wormley B, et al. Childhood adversity, monoamine A geneotype, and risk for conduct disorder. Arch Gen Psychiatry 2004;61:738–44.

[122] Huizinga D, Haberstick BC, Smolen A, et al. Childhood maltreatment, subsequent antisocial behavior, and the role of monoamine oxidase A genotype. Biol Psychiatry 2006;60(7):677–83.

[123] Kim-Cohen J, Caspi A, Taylor A, et al. MAOA, maltreatment, and gene-environment inter-action predicting children's mental health: new evidence and a meta-analysis. Mol Psychi-atry 2006;11(10):903–13.

[124] Livesley WJ. Behavioral and molecular genetic contributions to a dimensional classifica-tion of personality disorder. J Personal Disord 2005;19(2):131–55.

[125] Kendler KS. Reflections on the relationship between psychiatric genetics and psychiatric nosology. Am J Psychiatry 2006;163(7):1138–46.

Recent Advances in the Biological Study of Personality Disorders

Antonia S. New, MD[a,b,*], Marianne Goodman, MD[a,b],
Joseph Triebwasser, MD[a,b], Larry J. Siever, MD[a,b]

[a]The Mount Sinai School of Medicine, One Gustave L. Levy Place, Box 1217,
New York, NY 10029, USA
[b]The James J. Peters VA Medical Center, 130 West Kingsbridge Road, Bronx, NY 10468, USA

Research into the neurobiology of personality disorders had a slow start compared with studies of other psychiatric illnesses. This may be in part because personality disorders have traditionally been conceptualized as resulting from environmental factors, while axis I disorders have been viewed as having a "biological basis" [1]. The starting point for the investigation of the neurobiology of any psychiatric disorder often is the observation that a disorder is at least partially heritable. That is, inherited predispositions give rise to a vulnerability that, in conjunction with environmental factors, leads to the full presentation of disease. The two personality disorders for which there is the best evidence of familial transmission and heritability are borderline (BPD) and schizotypal (SPD) personality disorders. Evidence for familial transmission and heritability for BPD and SPD is undoubtedly one of the primary reasons that the vast majority of neurobiological research in personality disorders has focused on these two illnesses. In this review, we will therefore describe neurobiological models for BPD in detail and touch upon the neurobiology of SPD.

Family studies of BPD show that the first-degree relatives of probands with BPD are 10 times more likely to have been treated for BPD or a "BPD-like personality disorder" [2], and affective instability and impulsivity were significantly more common in first-degree relatives of BPD patients, compared with other psychiatric probands. Family studies have also demonstrated an increased risk for SPD in family members of individuals with schizophrenia, which has led to the widely accepted view of SPD as part of the schizophrenia spectrum [3,4].

Family studies can indirectly reflect heritability; however, only twin studies provide definitive evidence for genetic heritability. Twin studies of BPD show substantial heritability scores of 0.65 to 0.76 [5–7]. Twin studies of SPD show that it too is highly heritable, although more variable in estimates of the

*Corresponding author. *E-mail address*: antonia.new@mssm.edu (A.S. New).

0193-953X/08/$ – see front matter   Published by Elsevier Inc.
doi:10.1016/j.psc.2008.03.011   psych.theclinics.com

proportion of the variance explainable by genetic factors (0.35 to 0.81) [7–10]. Studies of symptom dimensions suggest that the positive and negative components of schizotypy are relatively genetically independent, although each may be related to underlying cognitive disorganization [11].

BORDERLINE PERSONALITY DISORDER

Early work in BPD investigated neurochemical abnormalities, focusing specifically on promising discoveries implicating an abnormality in serotonergic transmission. In addition to serotonergic mechanisms, another line of work has explored abnormalities in opiate responsiveness, specifically as it relates to self-injurious behavior, a striking and disturbing symptom prevalent in BPD. Finally, recent work has moved away from strictly molecular and neurochemical studies into the examination of neural circuitry abnormalities in BPD with brain imaging studies. We will review these three lines of research.

Serotonergic System Findings

Neuroendocrine challenge and metabolite studies

An illness as complex as BPD most likely involves multiple neurotransmitter systems. Laboratory and treatment-response data about the disorder supports a role for dopaminergic [12,13] and adrenergic [14,15] dysfunction. However, the neurotransmitter domain of greatest interest in BPD has been and continues to be the serotonin (5-HT) system, the assumed site of action of the specific serotonin reuptake inhibitors (SSRIs), which have been shown to reduce anger [16] and mood instability [17,18] in patients with the disorder.

Interest in 5-HT's role in BPD was spurred by findings of decreased cerebrospinal fluid (CSF) concentrations of the 5-HT metabolite 5-hydroxyindoleacetic acid (5-HIAA) in BPD patients with suicidal behavior [19,20] and impulsive aggression [19], although it has since become clear that impulsive aggression is associated with decreased CSF 5-HIAA in a variety of clinical populations [21–27]. A series of studies have shown decreased serotonergic responsivity in impulsive aggression in personality disorders, by demonstrating blunted hormonal responses to pharmacologic stimulation of the 5-HT system, through the use of such agents as fenfluramine, *meta*-chloropiperazine (m-CPP) and flesinoxan [28–30]. Other studies of peripheral markers in BPD patients have demonstrated decreased platelet paroxetine binding compared with controls, perhaps reflecting presynaptic serotonergic dysfunction [31]. Research into decreased serotonergic responsiveness in BPD has since turned to brain-imaging studies to explore central serotonergic responsiveness more directly [32]; these studies are reviewed later in this article.

Genetic studies

Another body of evidence for serotonergic abnormalities in BPD has emerged from genetic association studies. Research into the specific genes in BPD is still at a very early stage, in part because, as in most psychiatric disorders, the heritable component of BPD almost undoubtedly consists of multiple genes of small effect. A recent case-control study showed a significant association between the 5-HTT gene and BPD, with higher frequencies of the 10 repeat of the intron 2 VNTR marker and the S-10 haplotype of the 5-HTT promoter region polymorphism (5-HTTLPR), and fewer 12 repeat and LA-12 haplotypes, in BPD patients compared with healthy controls [33], while a study in bulimic women found the S allele to be a significant predictor of BPD [34]. A simultaneous case-control study was unable to replicate these associations [35], although the same research group found correlations between 5-HTTLPR and intron 2 VNTR genotypes and personality trait variations within a BPD cohort, on measures including impulsivity and sensation seeking [36]. The 5-HTTLPR S allele has also been shown to predict poorer treatment response to flexible-dose fluoxetine in BPD, as measured by the Overt Aggression Scale–Modified [37].

Mechanistically, the 5-HTTLPR S allele gives rise to lower levels of transcription of the transporter, which in principle would lead to increased 5-HT concentration in the synaptic cleft. An association between the S allele and BPD would seem, then, to contradict the neuroendocrine findings of decreased serotonergic activity in patients with the disorder. While the true mechanism underlying this finding has yet to be elucidated, a possible explanation is that the effect of those genetic variants may be more pronounced during brain development [38–40], which could outweigh its direct effect on 5-HTT binding in adulthood [41].

Another gene that has been implicated in impulsive aggression and suicidal behavior, common features of BPD, is the tryptophan hydroxylase (TPH) gene. TPH is the first enzyme in 5-HT biosynthesis. Two isoforms are known, TPH-1 and TPH-2. TPH-1 has been correlated with various psychiatric and behavioral disorders by gene polymorphism association studies. A recent case-control study of 95 women with BPD and 98 healthy controls showed that one six-single-nucleotide polymorphism (SNP) haplotype was absent from the control group, while representing about one quarter of all haplotypes in the BPD group. A "sliding window" analysis attributed the strongest disease association to haplotype configurations located between the gene promoter and intron 3 [42]. Turning from 5-HT synthesis to 5-HT degradation, a recent case-control study found that BPD patients had a greater frequency of the high-activity monoamine oxidase A gene promoter VNTR allele than did healthy volunteers [43].

Other 5-HT-related genes that have been examined in BPD include that encoding the 5-HT2A receptor, a polymorphism of whose promoter region has been associated with variations in impulsivity in healthy volunteers [44]. A study of SNPs in the 5-HT2A receptor gene in suicide attempters and healthy volunteers found genetic correlations with suicidal behavior in general as well as with nonviolent and impulsive suicidal behavior, anger, and aggression [45]. A case-control study failed to find an association between any of four polymorphisms of this gene and BPD diagnosis itself, but did disclose associations within the cohort between higher extraversion and both the C allele of rs6313 and the A allele of rs4941573 [46].

Taken together, the published evidence suggests that there is an abnormality in serotonergic function that underlies the impulsive aggressive symptoms of BPD, and that this may be related to specific genetic risk factors, but the precise molecular nature of this abnormality is not yet clear.

Opiate Neurocircuitry Findings

A subset of BPD patients mutilates themselves; for many clinicians, habitual nonsuicidal self-mutilation in a noninstitutionalized adult is considered pathognomonic of this disorder. It seems reasonable, then, to wonder whether disturbances of endogenous opiate pathways constitute part of BPD's underlying pathophysiology.

There is evidence, for example, that dissociation, another hallmark of BPD, is linked to disturbances in the pain-processing system. BPD patients who engage in deliberate self-harm show evidence of diminished pain sensitivity [47,48], which tends to normalize with global clinical improvement [32]. Decreased pain sensitivity, in turn, is associated with dissociation [49], and the opioid receptor antagonist naltrexone has been successfully used in open-label trials to treat both dissociation [50] and deliberate self-harm [51–53]. Functional neuroimaging of pain processing in BPD implicates abnormal activity in limbic and prefrontal regions, which seems to occur in response not just to painful stimuli but to emotionally disturbing ones as well [32].

Disturbances in the pain-processing system may be the common link among such core BPD symptoms as physical self-destructiveness, impulsivity, and dissociation. Given the low CSF endogenous opiate levels seen in BPD patients (Barbara Stanley, personal communication, 2007) and the region-specific increases in mu opioid receptors seen in the brains of suicide victims [54], a primary underdevelopment of the endogenous opiate system may result in a secondary up-regulation of mu opioid receptors. This might explain both BPD patients' vulnerability to opiate use disorders [55] and to self-mutilation, which may constitute efforts to generate an "endorphin rush." Another component of the opioid circuitry of interest in BPD is the kappa receptor system, overactivity of which may be related to the depressive symptoms [56,57], depersonalization [58], and intermittent thought disturbance [59] seen in affected patients.

Neuroimaging in Borderline Personality Disorder

Orbital frontal cortex and anterior cingulate gyrus

The concept that prefrontal cortex (PFC) controls and inhibits amygdala and other limbic structures was proposed many years ago [60]. Preclinical data indicate that areas of PFC exert inhibitory control over emotional responses. Specifically, in primates, damage to lateral PFC causes a loss of inhibitory control in attention tasks [61,62], whereas damage to orbital frontal cortex (OFC) causes a loss of inhibitory control in "affective" processing and increased aggression [63]. Studies in human beings have also implicated OFC and ventral anterior cingulated gyrus (ACG) in the control of emotion and specifically in the control of aggressive behavior [64,65]. In addition, injury to OFC early in childhood can result in disinhibited, aggressive behavior later in life [66].

It is now widely accepted that PFC, particularly OFC and adjacent ventral medial cortex (including ACG), plays a central role in the regulation of aggression [67–70].

Structural. Anatomical magnetic resonance imaging (MRI) studies comparing BPD patients to healthy controls show significant volume reduction with manually traced assessment of right ACG (Brodmann area [BA] 24) and left OFC in BPD subjects [71], but this was not confirmed in a larger sample using voxel-based morphometry [72]. Recent work in a large sample of manually traced MRI scans showed specific reductions in *gray* matter volume in ACG (BA 24) in BPD subjects compared with controls [73], replicating in a larger sample the earlier finding of volume reduction in ACG.

Resting positron emission tomography. Two resting studies using 18-fluorodeoxyglucose positron emission tomography (^{18}FDG PET), showed decreased metabolism in patients with BPD compared with healthy volunteers in anterior and medial frontal regions (BA 9,10, 32, 46) [74,75]. Another ^{18}FDG PET study showed that BPD patients with depression had less relative uptake in ACG (BA 32) at baseline compared with depressed patients without BPD [76]. In contrast, one resting PET study showed increased metabolism in female patients with BPD in frontal and ACG regions (BA 32, 8, 10) [77].

Serotonergic studies. Peripheral evidence for decreased serotonergic responsiveness in BPD led to brain imaging studies to explore central serotonergic responsiveness more directly. A number of studies have demonstrated decreased metabolic activity in OFC and ACG in response to serotonergic challenge in impulsive aggressive patients with BPD compared with healthy controls. One such study, using PET, found that while normal subjects showed increased metabolism in OFC and ACG following d,l-fenfluramine, impulsive aggressive patients with personality disorders showed significant increases only in inferior parietal lobe [78]. A larger study confirming prefrontal hypometabolism in response to d,l-fenfluramine demonstrated that healthy controls show increased metabolism in ACG and OFC following serotonergic stimulation, while BPD patients show decreased metabolism in these areas [75]. Our work employing ^{18}FDG PET to assess relative metabolic activity after m-CPP administration showed reduced metabolic responses in medial OFC and ACG in impulsive aggressive patients, all but one of whom met criteria for BPD, compared with controls [79]. In addition, we showed increased activity in posterior cingulate both at rest and in response to a serotonergic challenge; posterior cingulate is a brain area that has been specifically implicated in the recognition of facial emotion and therefore is particularly interesting in BPD [80,81]. Further support for serotonergically mediated hypometabolism in OFC in BPD comes from evidence of a normalization of OFC function with fluoxetine treatment in impulsive-aggressive BPD patients [82].

The mechanism of the serotonergic abnormality in BPD has been examined more closely with molecular neuroimaging studies. A PET study of 5-HT synthesis showed lower synthesis in men with BPD compared with controls in medial frontal gyrus, ACG, superior temporal gyrus, and corpus striatum; women with BPD had lower 5-HT synthesis compared with controls in right ACG and superior temporal gyrus [83]. More recently, we employed the 5-HTT PET radiotracer [11C]McN5652 to show reduced availability of 5-HTT in ACG of personality disordered individuals with impulsive aggression compared with healthy controls, suggesting reduced serotonergic innervation in this brain region [84]. A single-photon emission computed tomography (SPECT) study using [I-123] ADAM noted, in BPD subjects, 43% higher ADAM binding in the brainstem and 12% higher binding in the hypothalamus, suggesting increased levels of brain serotonin transporter availability [85]. Moreover, the ADAM binding correlated with levels of impulsivity. These findings lend further support to serotonergic dysfunction in BPD.

PET challenge studies. While the strongest case for a deficit in serotonin-mediated activation of OFC and ACG has been made in BPD patients selected for impulsive aggression, poor emotion regulation is a closely related symptom cluster. Indeed, the same brain regions that modulate the expression of aggression and anger have been implicated in the control of fear and other emotions [86–88], and affective instability is highly correlated with impulsive aggression in BPD [89–91].

Use of $[^{15}O]H_2O$ PET permits the measurement of regional brain blood flow under various conditions. This approach has been employed using script-driven imagery of abandonment in BPD and healthy controls during tracer uptake. Memories of abandonment were associated with underactivity of OFC, greater increases in blood flow in dorsolateral prefrontal cortex (DLPFC) and greater decreases in right ACG in women with BPD than in controls [92]. It should be noted, however, that most subjects in the BPD group were on psychoactive medications, while most in the control group were not. Using script-driven imagery of child abuse during PET, women with child abuse histories but not BPD showed increased blood flow in right DLPFC, right ACG, and left OFC, but decreased blood flow in left DLPFC, while women with child abuse histories and BPD failed to activate these regions. In this study, too, most BPD subjects were on psychoactive medications, while most in the control group were not [48].

Functional magnetic resonance imaging. Functional magnetic resonance imaging (fMRI) provides the opportunity for more finely grained time-resolution of brain activation during specific tasks through event-related designs. While this approach has been used widely in the study of mental illnesses such as posttraumatic stress disorder (PTSD) and depression, such work is still in its early phases in BPD. Consistent with theories of diminished activity in regions modulating emotional responses, a recent study showed that in response to angry faces, BPD patients exhibited attenuated activation in ACG compared with controls [93]. In one study, BPD subjects displayed increased blood oxygen level-dependent (BOLD) responses in bilateral OFC and insular regions, in left ACG and medial PFC compared with controls in response to emotional pictures [94]. Interestingly, a small pilot study (BPD, n = 6) showed that treatment with Dialectical Behavior Therapy (DBT) decreased response to negative pictures in right ACG, perhaps reflecting treatment-related attenuation of emotional responsiveness to unpleasant stimuli [95]. When subjected to painful heat stimuli during fMRI [96], BPD patients showed stronger activation in DLPFC and stronger deactivation in perigenual ACG.

In a recent study of Intermittent Explosive Disorder (IED), a phenotype that overlaps BPD in important respects, relative to controls, individuals with IED exhibited exaggerated amygdala reactivity and diminished OFC activation to angry faces. Furthermore, unlike controls, aggressive subjects failed to demonstrate amygdala-OFC coupling during responses to angry faces [97].

Amygdala
Early work viewed amygdala as the seat of fear, and an enormous amount of research has demonstrated this in rodents [98]. However, it has become clear in human studies that amygdala has a much more complex role to play. Amygdala can be activated equally when encoding both positive and negative emotions [99], and is involved more broadly in emotion inhibition and regulation [100] than was first apparent.

Structural. An early MRI study showed that total amygdala volume tended to be reduced in female BPD subjects compared with controls [101]. This was viewed as perhaps reflecting excitotoxicity with volume loss. Two subsequent small studies reported significant decreases in amygdala volume in BPD [71,102], although another study showed no difference in amygdala volume between BPD women and controls [103]. Two recent studies with much larger samples showed no difference in amygdala volume in BPD compared with controls [104,105]. Taken together, structural imaging studies lend support to a loss of volume in ACG (BA 24) in BPD but do not converge into a consistent finding of decreased amygdala volume.

Functional magnetic resonance imaging. A pilot study using exposure to standardized negative emotional images from the International Affective Picture System (IAPS) found increased activity in amygdala in six BPD patients compared with controls, which was interpreted as suggesting a neural substrate for the heightened emotional responsiveness seen in BPD [106]. In a study using affective versus neutral images from the Thematic Apperception Test, BPD subjects failed to show the differential response to emotional versus neutral pictures in amygdala, OFC, and ACG seen in healthy controls; this suggests that individuals with BPD may be equally emotionally responsive to neutral and to emotional stimuli. The authors did not examine group differences in BOLD response to neutral pictures alone.

Specific investigations of regional brain activity in response to emotional faces in BPD have shown overactivation of amygdala to faces, regardless of emotional valence, compared with a fixation point, and postscan debriefing revealed that some BPD patients had difficulty disambiguating neutral faces or found them threatening [107]. In a recent study with emotional faces, BPD subjects showed significantly greater activation than controls to fearful compared with neutral faces in right amygdala [93].

Connectivity studies. More recently, the tight coupling of metabolic activity between OFC and amygdala, specifically ventral amygdala, seen in healthy subjects was shown to be absent in BPD patients with impulsive aggression [105]. This raises the possibility that differential connectivity among brain regions may underlie abnormal aggression modulation in BPD, and that brain regions such as ACG [108] that normally modulate expressions of anger fail to come on line in BPD when needed. These findings further support the model of an over-reading of emotion in borderline patients and of deficits in activity in brain regions central to "top-down" modulation of emotional responses.

Hippocampus
The hippocampus, located in the medial temporal lobe, is involved in memory, and several reports have suggested its involvement in BPD. Hippocampal volume reduction was noted in three separate studies of female BPD subjects with histories of early traumatization [101,102,109]. Additionally, reduced hippocampal gray matter volume was noted in BPD subjects, and hippocampal volume was inversely correlated with lifetime aggressive behavior but not impulsivity [110].

Other regions
The posterior cingulate cortex is the backmost part of the cingulate cortex and has been specifically implicated in the recognition of facial emotion and therefore is particularly interesting in BPD [80,81]. The insular cortex has become a focus of attention because of its involvement in subjective emotional experience and body representation and its purported role in producing emotionally relevant context for sensory experience. It is important in the experience of pain and in basic emotions such as anger, joy, and disgust.

In the m-CPP study referred to earlier [79], increased metabolic activity was also seen in BPD subjects in posterior cingulate both at rest and in response to m-CPP. Treatment with DBT in a small pilot study decreased response to negative pictures in posterior cingulate cortices as well as in left insula [95]. In a study exploring individualized autobiographical memories of unresolved and resolved negative life events, when contrasting the former with the latter, patients, but not healthy subjects, showed activation in the regions delineated in this article so far: insula, amygdala, ACG and left posterior cingulate cortex. However additional regions were activated in patients, including the right occipital cortex, bilateral cerebellum, and midbrain [111].

Finally, a recent study demonstrated under-activity in the insula in BPD in response to unpleasant pictures [112] (Table 1). Although not specifically remarked on by the authors, this finding might be specifically interesting in relation to the interpersonal difficulties in BPD. There are a group of neurons called "mirror" or "Von Economo" neurons, which are present only in great apes and in human beings, and with greater abundance in human beings than in any other species [113,114]. These neurons have been implicated in perception of emotion and pain in others; they were first described as a network activated both during the observation of a motor action as well as during the execution of the same action [115]. It has become clear that this "mirroring" phenomenon is not just present for observation of motor behavior but is also important in more complex behaviors; indeed, human studies have shown that specific brain regions are activated by subjects not only when they feel an emotion, but also when they observe the same emotion in others. This holds true for the experience of physical pain [116] as well as for the observation of facial expressions of pain [117], and has been viewed as the neural substrate for "empathy." Von Economo neurons are located in anterior insula and ACG [118]. fMRI studies have explored the specific brain regions activated in the replication of emotional experiences from one person to another, and have found activation of the frontal insula and dorsal ACG (the same regions in which the Von Economo neurons are located) [117,119–121]. These same brain regions are also activated in response to seeing someone one loves [122], in facial emotion recognition [114] and in mothers viewing images of their own children compared with other children [123]. Further work on insula responsiveness in BPD is clearly needed.

In summary, brain-imaging studies have provided evidence for disruption of the neural circuitry in brain areas known to underlie impulsive aggression and affective regulation in BPD. The published evidence suggests the presence of abnormalities in both the structure and function of areas of PFC, particularly OFC and adjacent ventral medial cortex (including ACG), brain regions that underlie the modulation of emotional responses in BPD. The precise molecular nature of this abnormality remains unclear. Additional questions to be answered include whether BPD also involves a primary hyperactivity of the amygdala or a disconnection between regulatory regions and the amygdala. The role of other brain regions including insula and posterior cingulated, are being clarified and will undoubtedly increase our understanding of this complex disease.

Future Directions in BPD Research

Surprisingly little is known about the childhood and adolescent antecedents of adult BPD. Also, much of what we do know is based on data obtained retrospectively from adult borderlines, which is subject to the "negative halo" recall bias inevitable with already ill probands [124]. This bias may be especially pronounced in BPD patients who, as a group, may be highly prone to cast a negative emotional tone over memories of prior experiences and interactions, possibly distorting the accuracy of the memories [125]. A future direction of study will be to define prospectively the childhood and adolescent clinical features associated with adult BPD, as well as more rigorously to characterize the "borderline syndromes" of youth.

Table 1
Summary of brain imaging findings in BPD

Symptom/syndrome targeted	Modality	Brain area
Orbital Frontal Cortex/Cingulate Gyrus		
BPD	Structural MRI	↓ volume left OFC and right ACG (BA 24) [71]
BPD		↓ gray matter volume ACG (BA 24) [73]
BPD		↓ left ACG gray matter concentration (BA 24) [155]
BPD	Serotonergic PET	↓ metabolism in response to fenfluramine widely in frontal cortex including OFC [75]
Aggressive cluster BPDs		↓ metabolism in response to fenfluramine in OFC and ACG [78]
BPD		Men: ↓ 5-HTT synthesis in medial frontal gyrus, ACG, superior temporal gyrus, and corpus striatum. Women: ↓ 5-HTT synthesis in right ACG, superior temporal gyrus [83].
Aggressive cluster BPDs		↓ metabolism in response to m-CPP in OFC and ACG, increased in posterior cingulate [79]
BPD		Activation of OFC in response to fluoxetine [82]
Aggressive cluster BPDs		↓ 5-HTT density in ACG compared with controls [84]
BPD-IED		decreased coupling of resting metabolism between OFC and ventral ACG [105]
BPD	fMRI	More ACG BOLD response to facial fear but not anger compared with controls [155]
BPD		Less activation to pain and higher pain threshold than controls. Patients more active in DLPFC and less in ACG and ventromedial PFC in response to abandonment scripts [96].
BPD		Less activation to pain and higher pain threshold than controls. Patients more active in DLPFC and deactivated in ACG in response to pain [96].
BPD		Patients activated insula and ACC in response to "unresolved" more than "resolved" life events compared with controls [111]
BPD		↓ BOLD response to unpleasant pictures in ACG and left insula than controls [94]

	Method	Findings
Amygdala		
BPD	Structural MRI	Smaller amygdala volume and increase of amygdala creatine concentrations in BPD [156]
BPD ± MDD		↓ amygdala volume with MDD, but not in BPD without MDD [104]
BPD-IED		No difference in amygdala patients versus controls [105]
BPD	fMRI	More amygdala regardless of emotional expression than controls [107]
BPD		Patients deactivated in amygdala in response to pain [96]
BPD		Patients activated amygdala to "unresolved" more than "resolved" life events compared with controls [111]
BPD		Less amygdala BOLD response to facial fear but not anger compared with controls [93]
Hippocampus		
BPD with PTSD	Structural MRI	↓ hippocampal volume, correlated with extent of trauma [109]
BPD		↓ hippocampal volume, correlated with aggression [110]
BPD with childhood abuse		↓ hippocampal volume correlated with abuse [103]
BPD	PET	↑ 5-HT2A receptor in hippocampus [157]
Other regions/White matter		
BPD		↓ resting metabolism in temporal and medial parietal cortex [158]
BPD		Metabolism in response to fenfluramine: Males: ↓ in parietal and occipital cortex; Females: ↓ in temporal cortex [159]
BPD	White matter tracts	Corpus callosum not different from controls [160]
BPD		DTI in inferior frontal white matter not different from controls [161]
BPD + ADHD		DTI in inferior frontal white matter microstructural abnormalities seen in BPD + ADHD [161]

Abbreviations: ACG, anterior cingulate gyrus; ADHD, attention-deficit disorder hyperactivity disorder; BA, Brodmann area; BOLD, blood oxygenation level; BPD, borderline personality disorder; DLPFC, dorsolateral prefrontal cortex; DTI, diffusion tensor imaging; 5-HTT, serotonin transporter; fMRI, functional MRI; IED, intermittent explosive disorder; m-CPP, meta-chloropiperazine; MDD, major depressive disorder; OFC, orbital frontal cortex; PCG, posterior cingulate gyrus; PDs, personality disorders; PET, positron emission tomography; PTSD, posttraumatic stress disorder.

Almost nothing is known empirically about the clinical course of the disorder as afflicted individuals become elderly. The longest naturalistic longitudinal study followed patients over 27 years into middle age and found an attenuation of symptoms in a group of patients as the mean age reached 50 years, especially in symptoms related to disturbed interpersonal relationships [126]. Similarly, a 10-year follow-up study of a group of borderline patients found high rates of remission in a group whose mean age at follow-up was in the mid-30s [127]. The lack of information about *geriatric* BPD, however, is in striking contradistinction to our knowledge about late-life depression, which has been the focus of extensive phenomenological and therapeutic investigation. Clinical teaching has suggested that some of the most severe impulsive symptoms of BPD attenuate in late life, but no systematic research has demonstrated this. The best longitudinal data in BPD has tracked individuals from early adulthood to early middle age, but beyond that is unknown territory. Our clinical experience suggests that this disorder persists as a source of severe symptoms and functional impairment into late life. Tracking the disorder over the lifespan will provide the opportunity to look for clinical and biological predictors of the course of BPD.

Another important direction for future research will be the exploration of the neurobiology of interpersonal dysfunction in BPD. Only recently have there been neurobiological models of social interactions. Recent work in rodents defining the long-term neurobiological consequences of maternal care is one such example of new advances in the neurobiology of social interaction (reviewed in Zhang and colleagues [128]). Further work on the insula and mirror neuron activity in BPD will clearly be important, as noted above. Finally, an important role for the neuropeptides, oxytocin and vasopressin, in social attachment is clear (reviewed by Insel and Young [129]). These peptides are involved in maternal and pair bonding and might have a role in the treatment of BPD, as the nature of the abnormalities in social attachment in BPD become better defined and understood.

SCHIZOTYPAL PERSONALITY DISORDER

Schizotypal personality disorder (SPD) is the most widely studied of the schizophrenia (SCZ) spectrum disorders; affected individuals evince signs and symptoms [130] and cognitive deficits [131] that resemble attenuated versions of corresponding features of SCZ itself. First detected as eccentricity and/ or low functioning in nonpsychotic biological relatives of SCZ patients [132], SPD is seen more frequently in biological offspring of mothers with than those without SCZ spectrum disorders [133] and has been shown by the Danish Adoption Study to be genetically related to SCZ [134] but not to psychotic affective disorders or to major depression or anxiety disorders [135]. However, a study that assessed offspring of probands with schizophrenic, affective, or no psychiatric disorders respectively found no difference in the rates of moderate-to-high numbers of SPD traits in the offspring of the two patient groups [136].

SPD patients demonstrate clinical and treatment response characteristics similar to, although less marked than, those of SCZ patients [137]. Also, there appears to be a pattern of cognitive impairment specific to the SCZ spectrum [138] that may center on disturbances in working memory [139] and may reflect relatively greater involvement of left hemisphere [140]. For these reasons, SPD has come to be viewed as an important window onto SCZ that may help shed light on the latter disorder's genetics and pathophysiology [141]. Unlike SCZ patients, SPD patients usually can be assessed and studied without the confounds of medication use, active psychosis, and substance-related disorders that can render functional neurobiological findings in SCZ difficult to interpret. Commonalities between SPD and SCZ patients on cognitive tests and on various neurophysiological measures, including eye-tracking abnormalities [142,143], sensory gating deficits [144], and impaired startle prepulse inhibition [145] may represent endophenotypes—quantifiable features associated with SCZ spectrum disorders that are more closely related than the clinical phenotypes to the disorders' genetic underpinnings [146].

SPD's relationship with SCZ can be studied not just with regard to features the two disorders have in common but also with regard to ways in which SPD and SCZ differ. Combined understanding of both the similarities and differences between SCZ and SPD may yield information concerning why SPD patients have the deficits they do as well why they are spared the frank hallucinations, elaborated delusions, and global psychosocial decline of SCZ. Thus, on many neurobiological measures, eg, sizes of the left anterior and temporal horns [147] and posterior corpus callosum [148], and metabolic rates in lateral temporal regions after a serial learning task [149], SPD patients show values intermediate between SCZ patients and healthy controls. However, in some neurobiological variables (eg, shape of the right mediodorsal nucleus region [150]; size of the genu of the corpus callosum; width of a region of the corpus callosum just posterior to the genu [148]; and medial frontal, medial temporal, and putamen glucose metabolic rates after a serial verbal learning task [151]), SPD, but not SCZ, patients show abnormalities, while in other variables (eg, putamen size [151] and HPA axis activation in response to 2-deoxyglucose [152]), SPD and SCZ patients show abnormalities in opposite directions. In general, there may be a pattern of temporal volume reductions in both SCZ and SPD but relative preservation of frontal lobe volume in SPD [153] as well as reduced striatal dopaminergic activity in SPD compared with SCZ [154]. Neurobiological findings such as these that distinguish SPD from SCZ may represent factors that protect SPD patients from SCZ's psychosis and catastrophic decline in functioning despite these individuals' vulnerability to cognitive-perceptual and interpersonal disturbance.

SUMMARY

While it is premature to provide a simple model for the vulnerability to the development of either BPD or SPD, it is clear that these heritable disorders lend themselves to fruitful neurobiological exploration. The most promising findings in BPD suggest that a diminished top-down control of affective responses, which is likely to relate to deceased responsiveness of specific midline regions of prefrontal cortex, may underlie the affective hyperresponsiveness in this disorder. In addition, genetic and neuroendocrine and molecular neuroimaging findings point to a role for serotonin in this affective disinhibition. It is also clear that SPD falls within the schizophrenia spectrum, but precisely the nature of what predicts full-blown schizophrenia as opposed to the milder symptoms of SPD is not yet clear.

References

[1] Siever LJ, Davis KL. A psychobiological perspective on the personality disorders. Am J Psychiatry 1991;148(12):1647–58.

[2] Loranger AW, Oldham JM, Tulis EH. Familial transmission of DSM-III borderline personality disorder. Arch Gen Psychiatry 1982;39(7):795–9.

[3] Kendler KS, Neale MC, Walsh D. Evaluating the spectrum concept of schizophrenia in the Roscommon Family Study. Am J Psychiatry 1995;152(5):749–54.

[4] Kendler KS, Gardner CO. The risk for psychiatric disorders in relatives of schizophrenic and control probands: a comparison of three independent studies. Psychol Med 1997;27(2):411–9.

[5] Torgersen S, Lygren S, Oien PA, et al. A twin study of personality disorders. Compr Psychiatry 2000;41(6):416–25.

[6] Ji WY, Hu YH, Huang YQ, et al. [A twin study of personality disorder heritability]. Zhonghua Liu Xing Bing Xue Za Zhi 2006;27(2):137–41 [in Chinese].

[7] Coolidge FL, Thede LL, Jang KL. Heritability of personality disorders in childhood: a preliminary investigation. J Personal Disord 2001;15(1):33–40.

[8] Kendler KS, Czajkowski N, Tambs K, et al. Dimensional representations of DSM-IV cluster A personality disorders in a population-based sample of Norwegian twins: a multivariate study. Psychol Med 2006;36(11):1583–91.

[9] Kendler KS, Myers J, Torgersen S, et al. The heritability of cluster A personality disorders assessed by both personal interview and questionnaire. Psychol Med 2007;37(5): 655–65.

[10] Lin CC, Su CH, Kuo PH, et al. Genetic and environmental influences on schizotypy among adolescents in Taiwan: a multivariate twin/sibling analysis. Behav Genet 2007;37(2): 334–44.

[11] Linney YM, Murray RM, Peters ER, et al. A quantitative genetic analysis of schizotypal personality traits. Psychol Med 2003;33(5):803–16.

[12] Friedel RO. Dopamine dysfunction in borderline personality disorder: a hypothesis. Neuropsychopharmacology 2004;29(6):1029–39.

[13] Joyce PR, McHugh PC, McKenzie JM, et al. A dopamine transporter polymorphism is a risk factor for borderline personality disorder in depressed patients. Psychol Med 2006;36(6): 807–13.

[14] Philipsen A, Richter H, Schmahl C, et al. Clonidine in acute aversive inner tension and self-injurious behavior in female patients with borderline personality disorder. J Clin Psychiatry 2004;65(10):1414–9.

[15] Simeon D, Knutelska M, Smith L, et al. A preliminary study of cortisol and norepinephrine reactivity to psychosocial stress in borderline personality disorder with high and low dissociation. Psychiatry Res 2007;149(1–3):177–84.

[16] Salzman C, Wolfson AN, Schatzberg A, et al. Effect of fluoxetine on anger in symptomatic volunteers with borderline personality disorder. J Clin Psychopharmacol 1995;15(1):23–9.

[17] Coccaro EF, Kavoussi RJ. Fluoxetine and impulsive aggressive behavior in personality disordered subjects. Arch Gen Psychiatry 1997;54:1081–8.

[18] Kavoussi RJ, Liu J, Coccaro EF. An open trial of sertraline in personality disordered patients with impulsive aggression. J Clin Psychiatry 1994;55(4):137–41.

[19] Brown GL, Ebert MH, Goyer PF, et al. Aggression, suicide, and serotonin relationships to CSF amine metabolites. Am J Psychiatry 1982;139:741–6.

[20] Gardner DL, Lucas PB, Cowdry RW. CSF metabolites in borderline personality disorder compared with normal controls. Biol Psychiatry 1990;28:247–54.

[21] Linnoila M, DeJong J, Virkkunen M. Family history of alcoholism in violent offenders and impulsive fire setters. Arch Gen Psychiatry 1989;46:613–6.

[22] Linnoila M, Virkkunen M, George T, et al. Serotonin, violent behavior and alcohol. In: Jansson B, Jornvall H, Rydberg U, editors. Toward a molecular basis of alcohol use and abuse. Switzerland: Birkhauser Verlag Base; 1994. p. 155–64.

[23] Virkkunen M, Rawlings R, Tokola R, et al. CSF biochemistries, glucose metabolism, and diurnal activity rhythms in alcoholic violent offenders, fire setters, and healthy volunteers. Arch Gen Psychiatry 1994;51(1):20–7.

[24] Stanley B, Molcho A, Stanley M, et al. Association of aggressive behavior with altered serotonergic function in patients who are not suicidal. Am J Psychiatry 2000;157(4): 609–14.

[25] Lidberg L, Belfrage H, Bertilsson L, et al. Suicide attempts and impulse control disorder are related to low cerebrospinal fluid 5-HIAA in mentally disordered violent offenders. Acta Psychiatr Scand 2000;101(5):395–402.

[26] Roy A, Adinoff B, Linnoila M. Acting out hostility in normal volunteers: negative correlation with levels of 5-HIAA in cerebrospinal fluid. Psychiatry Res 1988;24:187–94.

[27] Traskman-Bendz L, Asberg M, Schalling D. Serotonergic function and suicidal behavior in personality disorders. Ann N Y Acad Sci 1986;487:168–74.

[28] Coccaro E, Siever L, Klar M, et al. Serotonergic studies in patients with affective and personality disorders. Arch Gen Psychiatry 1989;44:573–88.

[29] O'Keane V, Maloney E, O'Neil H, et al. Blunted prolactin response to d-fenfluramine in sociopathy. Evidence for subsensitivity of central serotonergic function. Br J Psychiatry 1992;160:643–6.

[30] Coccaro E, Kavoussi R, Oakes M, et al. 5HT2a/2c receptor blockade by amesergide fully attenuates prolactin response to d-fenfluramine challenge in physically healthy human subjects. Psychopharmacology (Berl) 1996;126(1):24–30.

[31] Ng Ying Kin NM, Paris J, Schwartz G, et al. Impaired platelet [3H]paroxetine binding in female patients with borderline personality disorder. Psychopharmacology (Berl) 2005;182(3):447–51.

[32] Schmahl C, Bremner JD. Neuroimaging in borderline personality disorder. J Psychiatr Res 2006;40(5):419–27.

[33] Ni X, Chan K, Bulgin N, et al. Association between serotonin transporter gene and borderline personality disorder. J Psychiatr Res 2006;40(5):448–53.

[34] Steiger H, Richardson J, Joober R, et al. The 5HTTLPR polymorphism, prior maltreatment and dramatic-erratic personality manifestations in women with bulimic syndromes. J Psychiatry Neurosci 2007;32(5):354–62.

[35] Pascual JC, Soler J, Barrachina J, et al. Failure to detect an association between the serotonin transporter gene and borderline personality disorder. J Psychiatr Res 2008;42(1): 87–8.

[36] Pascual J, Soler J, Baiget M, et al. Association between the serotonin transporter gene and personality traits in borderline personality disorder patients evaluated with Zuckerman-Kuhlman Personality Questionnaire (ZKPQ). Actas Esp Psiquiatr 2007;35(6):382–6.

[37] Silva H, Iturra P, Solari A, et al. Serotonin transporter polymorphism and fluoxetine effect on impulsiveness and aggression in borderline personality disorder. Actas Esp Psiquiatr 2007;35(6):387–92.

[38] Ansorge MS, Zhou M, Lira A, et al. Early-life blockade of the 5-HT transporter alters emotional behavior in adult mice. Science 2004;306(5697):879–81.

[39] Lauder JM. Ontogeny of the serotonergic system in the rat: serotonin as a developmental signal. Ann N Y Acad Sci 1990;600:297–313 [discussion: 314].

[40] Lovejoy EA, Scott AC, Fiskerstrand CE, et al. The serotonin transporter intronic VNTR enhancer correlated with a predisposition to affective disorders has distinct regulatory elements within the domain based on the primary DNA sequence of the repeat unit. Eur J Neurosci 2003;17(2):417–20.

[41] Parsey RV, Hastings RS, Oquendo MA, et al. Effect of a triallelic functional polymorphism of the serotonin-transporter-linked promoter region on expression of serotonin transporter in the human brain. Am J Psychiatry 2006;163(1):48–51.

[42] Zaboli G, Gizatullin R, Nilsonne A, et al. Tryptophan hydroxylase-1 gene variants associate with a group of suicidal borderline women. Neuropsychopharmacology 2006;31(9): 1982–90.

[43] Ni X, Sicard T, Bulgin N, et al. Monoamine oxidase A gene is associated with borderline personality disorder. Psychiatr Genet 2007;17(3):153–7.

[44] Nomura M, Kusumi I, Kaneko M, et al. Involvement of a polymorphism in the 5-HT2A receptor gene in impulsive behavior. Psychopharmacology (Berl) 2006;187(1):30–5.

[45] Giegling I, Hartmann AM, Moller HJ, et al. Anger- and aggression-related traits are associated with polymorphisms in the 5-HT-2A gene. J Affect Disord 2006;96(1–2):75–81.

[46] Ni X, Bismil R, Chan K, et al. Serotonin 2A receptor gene is associated with personality traits, but not to disorder, in patients with borderline personality disorder. Neurosci Lett 2006;408(3):214–9.

[47] Russ MJ, Roth SD, Lerman A, et al. Pain perception in self-injurious patients with borderline personality disorder. Biol Psychiatry 1992;32(6):501–11.

[48] Schmahl CG, Vermetten E, Elzinga BM, et al. A positron emission tomography study of memories of childhood abuse in borderline personality disorder. Biol Psychiatry 2004;55(7):759–65.

[49] Kemperman I, Russ MJ, Clark WC, et al. Pain assessment in self-injurious patients with borderline personality disorder. Psychiatry Res 1997;70(3):175–83.

[50] Bohus M, Landwehrmeyer GB, Stiglmayr C, et al. Naltrexone in the treatment of dissosciative symptoms in patients with borderline personality disorder. J Clin Psychiatry 1999;60: 598–603.

[51] Griengl H, Dantendorfer K. Naltrexone as a treatment of self-injurious behavior: a case report. Eur Psychiatry 2001;16(3):193–4.

[52] McGee MD. Cessation of self-mutilation in a patient with borderline personality disorder treated with naltrexone. J Clin Psychiatry 1997;58(1):32–3.

[53] Roth AS, Ostroff RB, Hoffman RE. Naltrexone as a treatment for repetitive self-injurious behaviour: an open-label trial. J Clin Psychiatry 1996;57(6):233–7.

[54] Gross-Isseroff R, Dillon KA, Israeli M, et al. Regionally selective increases in mu opioid receptor density in the brains of suicide victims. Brain Res 1990;530:312–6.

[55] Saper JR, Lake AE III. Borderline personality disorder and the chronic headache patient: review and management recommendations. Headache 2002;42(7):663–74.

[56] Kumor K, Su TP, Vaupel B, et al. Studies of kappa agonist. NIDA Res Monogr 1986;67: 18–25.

[57] Schlaepfer TE, Strain EC, Greenberg BD, et al. Site of opioid action in the human brain: mu and kappa agonists' subjective and cerebral blood flow effects. Am J Psychiatry 1998;155(4):470–3.

[58] Walsh SL, Strain EC, Abreu ME, et al. A selective kappa opioid agonist: comparison with butorphanol and hydromorphone in humans. Psychopharmacology (Berl) 2001;157(2): 151–62.

[59] Pfeiffer A, Brantl V, Herz A, et al. Psychotomimesis mediated by kappa opiate receptors. Science 1986;233(4765):774–6.

[60] McLean P. The limbic system ("visceral brain") and emotional behaviour. Arch Neurol Psychiatry 1955;73(2):130–4.

[61] Dias R, Robbins TW, Roberts AC. Dissociation in prefrontal cortex of affective and attentional shifts. Nature 1996;380(6569):69–72.

[62] Stefanacci L, Amaral DG. Some observations on cortical inputs to the macaque monkey amygdala: an anterograde tracing study. J Comp Neurol 2002;451(4):301–23.

[63] Izquierdo A, Suda RK, Murray EA. Comparison of the effects of bilateral orbital prefrontal cortex lesions and amygdala lesions on emotional responses in rhesus monkeys. J Neurosci 2005;25(37):8534–42.

[64] Davidson RJ, Putnam KM, Larson CL. Dysfunction in the neural circuitry of emotion regulation—a possible prelude to violence. Science 2000;289:591–4.

[65] Blair RJ. The roles of orbital frontal cortex in the modulation of antisocial behavior. Brain Cogn 2004;55(1):198–208.

[66] Anderson SW, Bechara A, Damasio H, et al. Impairment of social and moral behavior related to early damage in human prefrontal cortex. Nat Neurosci 1999;2:1032–7.

[67] Pribram KH, Bragshaw M. Further analysis of the temporal lobe syndrome utilizing frontotemporal ablation. J Comp Neurol 1953;99:347–75.

[68] Singh SD. Sociometric analysis of the effects of the bilateral lesion of frontal cortex on the social behavior of rhesus monkeys. Indian J Psychol 1976;51(2):144–60.

[69] Miller BL, Darby A, Benson DF, et al. Aggressive, socially disruptive and antisocial behaviour associated with fronto-temporal dementia. Br J Psychiatry 1997;170:150–4.

[70] Damasio H, Grabowski T, Frank R, et al. The return of Phineas Gage: clues about the brain from the skull of a famous patient. Science 1994;264:1102–5.

[71] Tebartz van Elst L, Hesslinger B, Thiel T, et al. Frontolimbic brain abnormalities in patients with borderline personality disorder: a volumetric magnetic resonance imaging study. Biol Psychiatry 2003;54(2):163–71.

[72] Rusch N, van Elst LT, Ludaescher P, et al. A voxel-based morphometric MRI study in female patients with borderline personality disorder. Neuroimage 2003;20(1):385–92.

[73] Hazlett EA, New AS, Newmark R, et al. Reduced anterior and posterior cingulate gray matter in borderline personality disorder. Biol Psychiatry 2005;58(8):614–23.

[74] De La Fuente JM, Goldman S, Stanus E, et al. Brain glucose metabolism in borderline personality disorder. J Psychiatr Res 1997;31(5):531–41.

[75] Soloff PH, Meltzer CC, Greer PJ, et al. A fenfluramine-activated FDG-PET study of borderline personality disorder. Biol Psychiatry 2000;47:540–7.

[76] Oquendo MA, Krunic A, Parsey RV, et al. Positron emission tomography of regional brain metabolic responses to a serotonergic challenge in major depressive disorder with and without borderline personality disorder. Neuropsychopharmacology 2005;30(6):1163–72.

[77] Juengling FD, Schmahl C, Hesslinger B, et al. Positron emission tomography in female patients with borderline personality disorder. J Psychiatr Res 2003;37(2):109–15.

[78] Siever LJ, Buchsbaum M, New A, et al. d,l- fenfluramine response in impulsive personality disorder assessed with 18F-deoxyglucose positron emission tomography. Neuropsychopharmacology 1999;20(5):413–23.

[79] New A, Hazlett E, Buchsbaum MS, et al. Blunted prefrontal cortical 18fluorodeoxyglucose positron emission tomography response to meta-chloropiperazine in impulsive aggression. Arch Gen Psychiatry 2002;59(7):621–9.

[80] Phillips ML, Bullmore ET, Howard R, et al. Investigation of facial recognition memory and happy and sad facial expression perception: an fMRI study. Psychiatry Res 1998;83(3):127–38.

[81] Sprengelmeyer R, Rausch M, Eysel UT, et al. Neural structures associated with recognition of facial expressions of basic emotions. Proc Biol Sci 1998;265(1409):1927–31.

[82] New AS, Buchsbaum MS, Hazlett EA, et al. Fluoxetine increases relative metabolic rate in prefrontal cortex in impulsive aggression. Psychopharmacology (Berl) 2004;176(3–4):451–8.

[83] Leyton M, Okazawa H, Diksic M, et al. Brain Regional alpha-[11C]methyl-L-tryptophan trapping in impulsive subjects with borderline personality disorder. Am J Psychiatry 2001;158(5):775–82.

[84] Frankle WG, Lombardo I, New A, et al. Brain serotonin transporter distribution in subjects with impulsive aggressivity: a positron emission study with [11C]McN 5652. Am J Pyschiatry 2005;162(5):915–23.

[85] Koch W, Schaaff N, Popperl G, et al. [I-123] ADAM and SPECT in patients with borderline personality disorder and healthy control subjects. J Psychiatry Neurosci 2007;32(4): 234–40.

[86] Orr SP, Metzger LJ, Lasko NB, et al. De novo conditioning in trauma-exposed individuals with and without posttraumatic stress disorder. J Abnorm Psychol 2000;109(2): 290–8.

[87] Peri T, Ben-Shakhar G, Orr SP, et al. Psychophysiologic assessment of aversive conditioning in posttraumatic stress disorder. Biol Psychiatry 2000;47(6):512–9.

[88] Anderson MC, Ochsner KN, Kuhl B, et al. Neural systems underlying the suppression of unwanted memories. Science 2004;303(5655):232–5.

[89] Sanislow CA, Grilo CM, McGlashan TH. Factor analysis of the DSM-III-R borderline personality disorder criteria in psychiatric inpatients. Am J Psychiatry 2000;157(10): 1629–33.

[90] Johansen M, Karterud S, Pedersen G, et al. An investigation of the prototype validity of the borderline DSM-IV construct. Acta Psychiatr Scand 2004;109(4):289–98.

[91] Fossati A, Madeddu F, Maffei C. Borderline personality disorder and childhood sexual abuse: a meta-analytic study. J Personal Disord 1999;13(3):268–80.

[92] Schmahl CG, Elzinga BM, Vermetten E, et al. Neural correlates of memories of abandonment in women with and without borderline personality disorder. Biol Psychiatry 2003;54(2):142–51.

[93] Minzenberg MJ, Fan J, New AS, et al. Fronto-limbic dysfunction in response to facial emotion in borderline personality disorder: an event-related fMRI study. Psychiatry Res 2007;155(3):231–43.

[94] Schnell K, Dietrich T, Schnitker R, et al. Processing of autobiographical memory retrieval cues in borderline personality disorder. J Affect Disord 2007;97(1–3):253–9.

[95] Schnell K, Herpertz SC. Effects of dialectic-behavioral-therapy on the neural correlates of affective hyperarousal in borderline personality disorder. J Psychiatr Res 2007;41(10): 837–47.

[96] Schmahl C, Bohus M, Esposito F, et al. Neural correlates of antinociception in borderline personality disorder. Arch Gen Psychiatry 2006;63(6):659–67.

[97] Coccaro EF, McCloskey MS, Fitzgerald DA, et al. Amygdala and orbitofrontal reactivity to social threat in individuals with impulsive aggression. Biol Psychiatry 2007;62(2): 168–78.

[98] LeDoux J. Emotion circuits in the brain. Annu Rev Neurosci 2000;23:155–84.

[99] Fitzgerald DA, Angstadt M, Jelsone LM, et al. Beyond threat: amygdala reactivity across multiple expressions of facial affect. Neuroimage 2006;30(4):1441–8.

[100] Phelps EA, LeDoux JE. Contributions of the amygdala to emotion processing: from animal models to human behavior. Neuron 2005;48(2):175–87.

[101] Driessen M, Herrmann J, Stahl K, et al. Magnetic resonance imaging volumes of the hippocampus and the amgydala in women with borderline personality disorder and early traumatization. Arch Gen Psychiatry 2000;57(12):1115–22.

[102] Schmahl CG, Vermetten E, Elzinga BM, et al. Magnetic resonance imaging of hippocampal and amygdala volume in women with childhood abuse and borderline personality disorder. Psychiatry Res 2003;122(3):193–8.

[103] Brambilla P, Soloff PH, Sala M, et al. Anatomical MRI study of borderline personality disorder patients. Psychiatry Res 2004;131(2):125–33.

[104] Zetzsche T, Frodl T, Preuss UW, et al. Amygdala volume and depressive symptoms in patients with borderline personality disorder. Biol Psychiatry 2006;60(3):302–10.

[105] New AS, Hazlett EA, Buchsbaum MS, et al. Amygdala-prefrontal disconnection in borderline personality disorder. Neuropsychopharmacology 2007;32(7):1629–40.

[106] Herpertz S, Dietrich T, Wenning B, et al. Evidence of abnormal amygdala functioning in borderline personality disorder: a functional MRI study. Biol Psychiatry 2001;50(4): 292–8.

[107] Donegan NH, Sanislow CA, Blumberg HP, et al. Amygdala hyperreactivity in borderline personality disorder: implications for emotional dysregulation. Biol Psychiatry 2003;54(11): 1284–93.

[108] Pietrini P, Guazzelli M, Basso G, et al. Neural correlates of imaginal aggressive behavior assessed by positron emission tomography in healthy subjects. Am J Psychiatry 2000;157(11):1772–81.

[109] Irle E, Lange C, Sachsse U. Reduced size and abnormal asymmetry of parietal cortex in women with borderline personality disorder. Biol Psychiatry 2005;57(2):173–82.

[110] Zetzsche T, Preuss UW, Frodl T, et al. Hippocampal volume reduction and history of aggressive behaviour in patients with borderline personality disorder. Psychiatry Res 2007;154(2):157–70.

[111] Beblo T, Driessen M, Mertens M, et al. Functional MRI correlates of the recall of unresolved life events in borderline personality disorder. Psychol Med 2006;36(6):845–56.

[112] Schnell K, Dietrich T, Schnitker R, et al. Processing of autobiographical memory retrieval cues in borderline personality disorder. J Affect Disord 2007;97(1–3):253–9.

[113] Nimchinsky EA, Gilissen E, Allman JM, et al. A neuronal morphologic type unique to humans and great apes. Proc Natl Acad Sci U S A 1999;96(9):5268–73.

[114] Parr LA, Waller BM, Fugate J. Emotional communication in primates: implications for neurobiology. Curr Opin Neurobiol 2005;15(6):716–20.

[115] Rizzolatti G, Craighero L. The mirror-neuron system. Annu Rev Neurosci 2004;27: 169–92.

[116] Singer T, Seymour B, O'Doherty J, et al. Empathy for pain involves the affective but not sensory components of pain. Science 2004;303(5661):1157–62.

[117] Botvinick M, Jha AP, Bylsma LM, et al. Viewing facial expressions of pain engages cortical areas involved in the direct experience of pain. Neuroimage 2005;25(1):312–9.

[118] Allman JM, Watson KK, Tetreault NA, et al. Intuition and autism: a possible role for Von Economo neurons. Trends Cogn Sci 2005;9(8):367–73.

[119] de Vignemont F, Singer T. The empathic brain: how, when and why? Trends Cogn Sci 2006;10(10):435–41.

[120] Saarela MV, Hlushchuk Y, Williams AC, et al. The compassionate brain: humans detect intensity of pain from another's face. Cereb Cortex 2007;17(1):230–7.

[121] Jackson PL, Brunet E, Meltzoff AN, et al. Empathy examined through the neural mechanisms involved in imagining how I feel versus how you feel pain. Neuropsychologia 2006;44(5):752–61.

[122] Bartels A, Zeki S. The neural correlates of maternal and romantic love. Neuroimage 2004;21(3):1155–66.

[123] Leibenluft E, Gobbini MI, Harrison T, et al. Mothers' neural activation in response to pictures of their children and other children. Biol Psychiatry 2004;56(4):225–32.

[124] Paris J. The diagnosis of borderline personality disorder: problematic but better than the alternatives. Ann Clin Psychiatry 2005;17(1):41–6.

[125] Bailey JM, Shriver A. Does childhood sexual abuse cause borderline personality disorder? J Sex Marital Ther 1999;25(1):45–57.

[126] Paris J, Zweig-Frank H. A 27-year follow-up of patients with borderline personality disorder. Compr Psychiatry 2001;42(6):482–7.

[127] Zanarini M. Pharmacological treatment of borderline personality disorder: two 12-week randomized double-blind placebo-controlled trials. Paper presented at: NCDEU 46th Annual Meeting. Boca Rotan, Florida, June 14, 2006.

[128] Zhang TY, Bagot R, Parent C, et al. Maternal programming of defensive responses through sustained effects on gene expression. Biol Psychol 2006;73(1):72–89.

[129] Insel TR, Young LJ. The neurobiology of attachment. Nat Rev Neurosci 2001;2(2):129–36.

[130] Dickey CC, McCarley RW, Niznikiewicz MA, et al. Clinical, cognitive, and social characteristics of a sample of neuroleptic-naive persons with schizotypal personality disorder. Schizophr Res 2005;78(2–3):297–308.

[131] Matsui M, Sumiyoshi T, Kato K, et al. Neuropsychological profile in patients with schizotypal personality disorder or schizophrenia. Psychol Rep 2004;94(2):387–97.

[132] Kety SS, Rosenthal D, Wender PH, et al. Mental illness in the biological and adoptive families of adopted individuals who have become schizophrenic. Behav Genet 1976;6(3):219–25.

[133] Tienari P, Wynne LC, Laksy K, et al. Genetic boundaries of the schizophrenia spectrum: evidence from the Finnish Adoptive Family Study of Schizophrenia. Am J Psychiatry 2003;160(9):1587–94.

[134] Kendler KS, Gruenberg AM, Strauss JS. An independent analysis of the Copenhagen sample of the Danish adoption study of schizophrenia II. The relationship between schizotypal personality disorder and schizophrenia. Arch Gen Psychiatry 1981;38:982–7.

[135] Kendler KS. Schizophrenia genetics and dysbindin: a corner turned? Am J Psychiatry 2004;161(9):1533–6.

[136] Squires-Wheeler E, Skodol AE, Bassett A, et al. DSM-III-R schizotypal personality traits in offspring of schizophrenic disorder, affective disorder, and normal control parents. J Psychiatr Res 1989;23(3–4):229–39.

[137] Koenigsberg HW, Reynolds D, Goodman M, et al. Risperidone in the treatment of schizotypal personality disorder. J Clin Psychiatry 2003;64(6):628–34.

[138] Mitropoulou V, Harvey PD, Maldari LA, et al. Neuropsychological performance in schizotypal personality disorder: evidence regarding diagnostic specificity. Biol Psychiatry 2002;52(12):1175–82.

[139] Mitropoulou V, Harvey PD, Zegarelli G, et al. Neuropsychological performance in schizotypal personality disorder: importance of working memory. Am J Psychiatry 2005;162(10):1896–903.

[140] Voglmaier MM, Seidman LJ, Niznikiewicz MA, et al. Verbal and nonverbal neuropsychological test performance in subjects with schizotypal personality disorder. Am J Psychiatry 2000;157:787–93.

[141] Avila MT, Adami HM, McMahon RP, et al. Using neurophysiological markers of genetic risk to define the boundaries of the schizophrenia spectrum phenotype. Schizophr Bull 2003;29(2):299–309.

[142] Siever LJ, Keefe R, Bernstein DP, et al. Eye tracking impairment in clinically identified schizotypal personality disorder patients. Am J Psychiatry 1990;147:740–5.

[143] Thaker GK, Cassady S, Adami H, et al. Eye movements in spectrum personality disorders: comparison of community subjects and relatives of schizophrenic patients. Am J Psychiatry 1996;153(3):362–8.

[144] Cadenhead KS, Light GA, Geyer MA, et al. Sensory gating deficits assessed by the P50 event-related potential in subjects with schizotypal personality disorder. Am J Psychiatry 2000;157:55–9.

[145] Cadenhead KS, Geyer MA, Braff DL. Impaired startle prepulse inhibition and habituation in schizotypal patients. Am J Psychiatry 1993;150:1862–7.

[146] Siever LJ. Endophenotypes in the personality disorders. Dialogues Clin Neurosci 2005;7(2):139–51.

[147] Buchsbaum M, Yang S, Hazlett E, et al. Ventricular volume and assymetry in schizotypal personality disorder and schizophrenia assessed with magnetic resonance imaging. Schizophr Res 1997;27:45–53.

[148] Downhill JE, Buchsbaum MS, Wei TS, et al. Shape and size of the corpus callosum in schizophrenia and schizotypal personality disorder. Schizophr Res 2000;42:193–208.

[149] Buchsbaum MS, Nenadic I, Hazlett E, et al. Differential metabolic rates in prefrontal and temporal Brodmann areas in schizophrenia and schizotypal personality disorder. Schizophr Res 2002;54(1–2):141–50.

[150] Hazlett EA, Buchsbaum MS, Byne W, et al. Three-dimensional analysis with MRI and PET of the size, shape and function of the thalamus in the schizophrenia spectrum. Am J Psychiatry 1999;156:1190–9.

[151] Shihabuddin L, Buchsbaum MS, Hazlett EA, et al. Striatal size and glucose metabolic rate in schizotypal personality disorder and schizophrenia. Arch Gen Psychiatry 2001;58: 877–84.

[152] Mitropoulou V, Goodman M, Sevy S, et al. Effects of acute metabolic stress on the dopaminergic and pituitary-adrenal axis activity in patients with schizotypal personality disorder. Schizophr Res 2004;70(1):27–31.

[153] Kirrane RM, Siever LJ. New perspectives on schizotypal personality disorder. Curr Psychiatry Rep 2000;2:62–6.

[154] Siever LJ, Davis KL. The pathophysiology of schizophrenia disorders: perspectives from the spectrum. Am J Psychiatry 2004;161(3):398–413.

[155] Minzenberg MJ, Fan J, New AS, et al. Frontolimbic structural changes in borderline personality disorder. J Psychiatr Res 2007 Sep 6; [Epub ahead of print].

[156] Tebartz van Elst L, Ludaescher P, Thiel T, et al. Evidence of disturbed amygdalar energy metabolism in patients with borderline personality disorder. Neurosci Lett 2007;417(1): 36–41.

[157] Soloff PH, Price JC, Meltzer CC, et al. 5HT(2A) receptor binding is increased in borderline personality disorder. Biological Psychiatry 2007;62(6):580–7.

[158] Lange C, Kracht L, Herholz K, et al. Reduced glucose metabolism in temporo-parietal cortices of women with borderline personality disorder. Psychiatry Res 2005;139(2): 115–26.

[159] Soloff PH, Meltzer CC, Becker C, et al. Gender differences in a fenfluramine-activated FDG PET study of borderline personality disorder. Psychiatry Res 2005;138(3):183–95.

[160] Zanettini R, Antonini A, Gatto G, et al. Valvular heart disease and the use of dopamine agonists for Parkinson's disease. N Engl J Med 2007;356(1):39–46.

[161] Rusch N, Weber M, Il'yasov KA, et al. Inferior frontal white matter microstructure and patterns of psychopathology in women with borderline personality disorder and comorbid attention-deficit hyperactivity disorder. Neuroimage 2007;35(2):738–47.

The Neurobiology of Psychopathy

Andrea L. Glenn, MA[a],*, Adrian Raine, PhD[b]

[a]Department of Psychology, University of Pennsylvania, 3809 Walnut Street, PA 19104, USA
[b]Departments of Criminology, Psychiatry, and Psychology, University of Pennsylvania, 3809 Walnut Street, PA 19104, USA

Psychopathy is a serious personality disorder characterized by emotional and behavioral abnormalities. The disorder is present in approximately 15% to 20% of criminal offenders [1] and is one of the strongest predictors of violent recidivism in prisoners [2]. Psychopaths tend to lack feelings of empathy, guilt, and remorse; they often lack fear of punishment, are impulsive, have difficulty regulating their emotions, and display antisocial and violent behavior. Psychopaths may use superficial charm, conning, and manipulation to take advantage of others. A unique feature of psychopathy is that, in addition to increased reactive aggression, they also display instrumental aggression [3]. Psychopathy encompasses a variety of personality and behavioral features, as demonstrated by the 20-item rating scale, the Psychopathy Checklist–Revised (PCL-R) [3], which has emerged as the gold standard for assessing psychopathy. The scale has traditionally been divided into two factors, with Factor 1 describing the interpersonal and affective features and Factor 2 describing socially deviant behaviors, although three- and four-factor models have also been proposed [3,4]; thus, it becomes clear that many of the features of psychopathy are relatively distinct and from different domains.

It is perhaps this "constellation" of features [5] that contribute to the seemingly widespread neurobiological deficits observed in psychopathy. Several brain-imaging studies have explored structural and functional differences in the brains of psychopaths, but very few have begun to look at the role of genetic factors or neurotransmitter and neuroendocrine functioning; thus, the field is still far from a molecular neuroscience account of psychopathy [6]. While psychopathy has thus far been found to be intransigent to treatment attempts [7], an understanding of the neural substrates of psychopathy will likely be a major contributor to future treatment and prevention.

NEUROTRANSMITTERS

In highly studied areas of psychopathology such as depression and schizophrenia, neurobiological research has advanced to the level of examining pathology

*Corresponding author. E-mail address: aglenn@sas.upenn.edu (A.L. Glenn).

0193-953X/08/$ – see front matter
doi:10.1016/j.psc.2008.03.004

at the level of neurotransmitter systems. To the authors' knowledge, only a few studies have examined the role of neurotransmitters in the development and maintenance of psychopathy. In two independent samples, Soderstrom and colleagues [8,9] found that psychopathy was associated with an increased ratio between the dopamine metabolite homovanillic acid (HVA) and the serotonin metabolite 5-hydroxyindoleacetic acid (5-HIAA). This increased ratio is thought to be an indicator of impaired serotonergic regulation of dopamine activity, which results in the disinhibition of aggressive impulses. It is suggested that dopamine-modulating drugs, possibly in combination with serotonin reuptake inhibitors might be potential pharmacologic treatments for psychopathy.

Reciprocal relationships have been shown to exist between neurotransmitter and endocrine systems. For example, serotonin neurotransmission has an effect on the hypothalamic-pituitary-adrenal (HPA) axis, so that increased activity at serotonin receptor sites in the hypothalamus increase the production of cortisol. Sobczak and colleagues [10] found that disruption of serotonin neurotransmission disrupts cortisol reactivity to a stress-inducing speech task. Thus, dysregulation of serotonin in the brain may contribute to the low cortisol levels observed in psychopathy. However, evidence also suggests that cortisol can have an effect on serotonin transmission in the brain [11]. Given the interdependence of these systems, it becomes highly difficult to localize a specific system that contributes to psychopathic characteristics; it is likely that a complex pattern of brain activity is involved.

Serotonin may also interact with testosterone levels to increase the probability of violent aggression. Evidence suggests that low serotonin levels combined with high testosterone levels augment the rates and intensity of aggression [12]. A recent review of the literature suggests that elevated testosterone alone does not account for aggressive behavior, as it is often observed in successful athletes and businessmen who are not necessarily more violence-prone; testosterone is more strongly associated with dominance than aggression [13]. It is hypothesized that elevated testosterone levels encourage dominance-seeking behaviors, yet when an individual becomes frustrated in an attempt to achieve dominance, low serotonin levels may increase the likelihood of an aggressive response. Low serotonin levels have been associated with impulsive and highly negative reactions, and thus may increase the tendency for violent aggression [13].

While early evidence suggests that dysregulation of neurotransmitter systems may be involved in psychopathy, additional studies are needed to explore this relationship and its implications further. Because neurotransmitters can interact with neuroendocrine systems, as well as affect the functioning of certain brain regions, it is important to gain an understanding of the role they may play in the development and maintenance of psychopathy.

NEUROENDOCRINOLOGY

In an analysis of recent research, Van Honk and Schutter [14] propose that the underlying source of emotional deficits observed in psychopathy are a result of an imbalance of the hormones cortisol and testosterone. Cortisol is a glucocorticoid hormone that is released upon activation of the HPA axis. The role of cortisol is to mobilize the body's resources and to provide energy in times of stress [15]; it is also involved in potentiating the state of fear [16], sensitivity to punishment, and withdrawal behavior [17]. Testosterone is a product of the hypothalamic-pituitary-gonadal (HPG) axis and is associated with approach-related behavior, reward sensitivity, and fear reduction [18]. Testosterone and cortisol have been shown to have mutually antagonistic properties. Cortisol suppresses the activity of the HPG axis on all levels, diminishing testosterone production and inhibiting its effects [19]. In turn, testosterone inhibits activity of the HPA axis [20]. Van Honk and colleagues [21] have found that injections of testosterone reduce fearfulness, promote responding to angry faces [22], and shift the balance from punishment to reward sensitivity [23]. In the latter study, Van Honk and colleagues found that a single administration of testosterone led to disadvantageous decision making in the Iowa gambling task, with participants showing decreased sensitivity to punishment and increased sensitivity to reward; thus, by manipulating the balance between cortisol and testosterone, critical changes can be observed in an individual's decision-making behavior. Van Honk and Schutter [14] proposes that low levels of cortisol, accompanied by high levels of testosterone, might contribute to primary psychopathy.

A few studies have found relationships between cortisol and psychopathy. Holi and colleagues [24] measured serum cortisol levels in young adult male psychopathic offenders with a history of violence and found a negative correlation with psychopathy, although the sample size was small. Low salivary cortisol levels were also observed in adolescents with callous-unemotional traits, which are thought to be similar to psychopathic traits in adults [25]. In a study of undergraduates, O'Leary and colleagues [26] found that males scoring higher in psychopathy showed less cortisol reactivity to a social stress test than lower-scoring males.

While several studies have explored the link between testosterone and aggression, very few studies have examined the relation between testosterone levels and psychopathy specifically. Stalenheim and colleagues [27] found that testosterone levels were positively related to scores on Factor 2 of the PCL-R, although it is possible the results may be confounded by comorbid substance abuse and other psychiatric disorders. Loney and colleagues [25] examined testosterone levels in boys with callous-unemotional traits, which are thought to be analogous to psychopathic traits in adulthood, but found no effects. In other antisocial and aggressive groups, higher testosterone levels have been found in girls with conduct disorder [28], adolescent boys with externalizing behaviors [29], young criminals [30–32], and criminal women [33], and have been associated with a variety of antisocial behaviors including difficulties on the job, nonobservance of the law, marriage failures, drug use, alcohol abuse, and violent behaviors [34]. It remains unclear, however, whether high testosterone levels are present in psychopaths.

In addition to exploring cortisol and testosterone levels in psychopathy, future studies may also want to examine the distributions and sensitivity of different receptors. For example, depression has been associated with an increased ratio between two different types of cortisol receptors, and also with decreased sensitivity in one type of receptor. Thus, it may be important to explore different aspects of neuroendocrine functioning in psychopathy.

Hormones have an effect on behavior by inducing chemical changes in specific brain regions, thus affecting the likelihood of certain behavioral outcomes by modulating neural pathways. In addition, both neurotransmitters and hormones are expressed at early periods of neural development, so it is likely that they participate in the structural organization of the nervous system [13]. Several studies have found differences in the structure in specific brain regions and networks, yet the underlying factors that may cause or maintain these abnormalities remains unknown.

SUBCORTICAL BRAIN STRUCTURES

It has been argued that dysfunction in the amygdala is central to the pathology associated with psychopathy [35]. Specifically, impaired amygdala functioning disrupts the ability to form stimulus-reinforcement associations, hindering the individual from learning to associate their harmful actions with the pain and distress of others. The amygdala is also necessary for aversive conditioning and for enhancing attention to emotional stimuli, which facilitates empathy for victims [36]. Psychopathy is associated with deficits in aversive conditioning [37], fearful facial expression recognition [38], passive avoidance learning [39], and augmentation of the startle reflex by visual threat primes [40]. Each of these deficits has also been associated with lesions to the amygdala [41].

Brain-imaging studies of psychopathy have revealed structural and functional abnormalities in the amygdala. Reduced volume of the amygdala has been reported in a study of psychopathic individuals [42]. In several functional MRI (fMRI) studies, reduced activity in the amygdala has been associated with psychopathy during the processing of emotional stimuli [43], during fear conditioning [44,45], during a socially interactive game [46], and during an affect recognition task [47]. However, two studies have reported *increased* amygdala activation in antisocial individuals while viewing negative visual content [48] and during aversive conditioning [49].

The source of impaired functioning in subcortical structures such as the amygdala remains to be elucidated, but impairments likely occur early in life [6]. One possibility is that hormone imbalances prenatally or in early childhood affect the development of subcortical structures, and may continue to influence functioning into adulthood [14]. A major binding site for steroid hormones is in the amygdala. Here, hormones have been shown to affect gene transcription, and therefore have the ability to affect functioning by increasing or decreasing the probability of certain responses such as approach or withdrawal behavior in response to threat [17].

Genetic and neurotransmitter factors may also affect amygdala functioning. Blair [50] highlights a study showing that individuals who are homozygous for the long version of the serotonin transporter gene (5-HTTLPR) show significantly reduced amygdala responses to emotional expressions relative to those with the short-form polymorphism [51] and behavioral impairment on emotional learning tasks that depend on the amygdala [52]. The amygdala has many serotonergic inputs and thus may be sensitive to changes in serotonin transmission.

In addition to the amygdala, abnormalities have also been observed in other subcortical regions such as the hippocampus. Raine and colleagues [53] found asymmetries within the hippocampus in unsuccessful (convicted) psychopaths. Hippocampal dysfunction may result in affect dysregulation, poor contextual fear conditioning, and insensitivity to cues predicting capture. Atypical brain asymmetries are thought in part to reflect disrupted neurodevelopmental processes [54]. Brain asymmetries first appear during fetal development, but tend to decrease somewhat with age in healthy children [55]. Structural asymmetries in psychopaths may reflect an interruption to the normal developmental process. Lakkso and colleagues [56] found psychopathy to be negatively correlated with the volume of the posterior hippocampus. The hippocampus has dense interconnections to both the amygdala and prefrontal cortex, which have also been implicated in psychopathy, so it may have an effect on and be affected by the functioning in these structures.

CORTICAL BRAIN STRUCTURES

Raine and colleagues [57] observed an 11% reduction in prefrontal gray matter volume in a group of individuals with antisocial personality disorder compared with both normal and psychiatric control groups. Furthermore, the individuals with antisocial personality disorder showed reduced skin conductance activity during a social stress test, and those with particularly low prefrontal gray matter showed particularly reduced stress reactivity. This study supports evidence that prefrontal regions, in particular the orbitofrontal cortex, are involved in generating somatic states. Indeed, Van Honk and colleagues [58] provided further evidence for this by using repeated transcranial magnetic stimulation (rTMS) to inhibit the activity of the orbitofrontal cortex and found that it resulted in significant reductions in skin conductance responding.

An additional finding of reduced prefrontal gray matter in psychopathy was later observed in a group of unsuccessful psychopaths, demonstrating a 22.3% reduction in gray matter [59]. Two studies have shown reduced gray matter volumes specifically in the orbitofrontal cortex in antisocial individuals [60,61]. Functional imaging studies have observed reduced activity associated with psychopathy in the orbitofrontal cortex during fear conditioning [44,45] and during a socially interactive game [46]. The orbitofrontal cortex is associated with the anticipation of punishment and reward, response reversal during changing reinforcement contingencies, and social cognition in general [62,63]. Lesion studies have demonstrated that damage to the orbitofrontal cortex often results in pathologic lying, irresponsibility, promiscuous sexual behavior, shallow affect, and a lack of guilt or remorse [64], all of which are characteristics of psychopathy.

Several studies have observed *increased* activation in higher cognitive areas such as the dorsolateral prefrontal cortex during emotional tasks in psychopaths compared with controls [43,46,47,65]. It has been suggested that psychopaths may use more cognitive resources to process affective information than nonpsychopaths [43].

OTHER STRUCTURES

While abnormalities in the amygdala and orbitofrontal regions are the best replicated, psychopathy has also been associated with abnormalities in other regions. Reduced functioning in the anterior cingulate has been observed during fear conditioning [44,45], in criminal psychopaths during an affective memory task [43], and in processing of emotional information [48]. The anterior cingulate is closely connected with the amygdala and is involved in emotional processing. Deficits in the angular gyrus (posterior superior temporal gyrus) have been found in psychopathic and antisocial individuals during a semantic processing task [66] and functioning of the posterior cingulate, which may be involved in self-referencing and experiencing emotion, has been observed in an fMRI study of psychopaths [43]. Reduced functioning of the insula has been observed during fear conditioning [44,45]; the insula is thought to be involved in the emotional processing of anticipatory anxiety and awareness of threat stimuli and associated body states [67]. Kiehl [68] argues for a paralimbic system dysfunction of psychopathy. In a thorough review of the literature, Kiehl points out that the seemingly distinct regions implicated in psychopathy, including the amygdala, parahippocampal region, anterior superior temporal gyrus, insula, anterior and posterior cingulate, and the orbitofrontal cortex share similar cytoarchitecture and have been grouped together to form the "paralimbic system." It is acknowledged that it remains unknown how or when the abnormalities in these brain regions arise. Indeed, it is difficult to determine whether each region that has been found to be associated with psychopathy makes a unique contribution to the disorder, or whether reduced input from key regions such as the amygdala or orbitofrontal cortex results in reduced functioning in other areas that are highly connected to these regions.

CONNECTIVITY

In addition to the abnormal functioning observed in certain brain regions of psychopaths, some studies have also explored the connectivity between areas. Van Honk and Schutter [14] hypothesize that disruptions in the connectivity between subcortical and cortical regions may contribute to psychopathy. Such connectivity allows emotional information from subcortical regions such as the amygdala to provide input to cortical regions, which is important in guiding decision making and cognitive evaluation [69]. Connectivity between the amygdala and orbitofrontal cortex may be especially important in the generation of somatic markers. The orbitofrontal cortex receives emotional input from the amygdala and stores representations of certain events or stimuli so they can be retrieved later. If an individual then recalls or anticipates these events or stimuli, the orbitofrontal cortex triggers the somatic state. If connectivity between the amygdala and orbitofrontal cortex is disrupted, the orbitofrontal cortex will be unable to form representations, and feelings such as anticipatory fear of aversive events will not be generated [70]. Indeed, reduced connectivity between the orbitofrontal cortex and the amygdala has been associated with lower sensitivity to threat cues (Harm Avoidance) [71]. The orbitofrontal cortex is also involved in dictating emotion regulation through inhibitory connections to the amygdala and anterior cingulate [72]; therefore, poor connectivity between these regions would also result in reduced regulation of subcortical structures by prefrontal areas. This may contribute to the disinhibition and reactive aggression observed in psychopathy.

Van Honk and Schutter [14] argue that an imbalance between cortisol and testosterone reduces subcortico-cortical communication. Cortisol has been shown to increase the exchange of information between subcortical and cortical brain regions and strengthen cortical control over subcortical drives [73]. In contrast, testosterone administrations have been shown to reduce subcortical-cortical cross-talk [74]. Since the frontal cortical areas rely on subcortical areas for emotion-related information, it is argued that the decoupling results in cortical processing that is purely cognitive, and is thus cold and instrumental [14]. However, it remains to be seen whether connectivity between subcortical and cortical regions is disrupted in psychopathy.

In addition to subcortico-cortical connectivity, psychopaths may also exhibit impaired connectivity between the two hemispheres of the brain. Recently, Hiatt and Newman [75] found that the time required to transfer information from one hemisphere to the other is significantly prolonged in criminal psychopaths compared with criminal nonpsychopaths. This effect was more pronounced in right-handed response conditions, which are controlled by the left hemisphere. They suggest that impaired connectivity between hemispheres may cause functions primarily mediated by the left hemisphere (eg, approach behavior and language processing) to be relatively unmodulated by functions mediated predominantly by the right hemisphere (eg, behavioral inhibition and emotion processing) and vice versa. While this hypothesis remains to be tested, it may prove to be an important link in explaining several seemingly distinct phenomena observed in psychopathy. Further evidence for impaired connectivity between hemispheres comes from a structural imaging study by Raine and colleagues [76] that found increased volume of the corpus callosum in psychopathic individuals. The corpus callosum is the major connection between the two hemispheres. Future imaging studies may help to further our understanding of the connectivity between hemispheres in psychopaths. Diffusion tensor imaging (DTI) can be used to trace fiber pathways between hemispheres, while functional imaging may help to examine the relationships between functioning of interconnected regions.

DEVELOPMENT

Neurobiological abnormalities associated with psychopathy appear to be widespread throughout the brain. Research has come a long way in examining different structures or groups of structures and how their abnormal functioning might contribute to psychopathic characteristics, yet many unanswered questions remain. It remains unclear how structural and functional brain abnormalities, as well as hormone and neurotransmitter imbalances, originate. It is also unknown how different systems interact to maintain a particular pattern of brain functioning.

Research suggests that psychopathic features are present at an early age, with indicators of temperamental and psychophysiological differences being detected as early as age 3 in individuals who develop psychopathic traits in adulthood [77]. Furthermore, a growing body of evidence is suggesting that psychopathic traits are identifiable in childhood [78,79]. Such research suggests that neurobiological impairments occur very early in life.

TREATMENT

Taking into consideration the recent developments in understanding the neurobiology of psychopathy, it would be predicted that potential treatments could aim to increase the functioning of key brain regions. This might be achieved in a variety of ways, including pharmacological mechanisms that might alter neurotransmitter or endocrine balances, or techniques that might directly alter the functioning of certain brain regions. Van Honk and Schutter [14] have suggested that pharmacological therapies that would restore the homeostatic balance between cortisol and testosterone could potentially help to sensitize a psychopath's emotional responsiveness so that behavioral therapies that previously failed may gain efficacy. A method that might directly alter the functioning of certain brain regions is repetitive transcranial magnetic stimulation (rTMS), a noninvasive technique that is used to stimulate the brain using very strong, pulsed magnetic fields; this results in changes in cortical excitability in the stimulated area. While research using the technique is still in its infancy, rTMS has been studied as a potential treatment for affective disorders, particularly depression, and in some cases has demonstrated results superior to placebo [80]. Depression has been associated with *increased* activity in the orbitofrontal cortex [81]. In a sample of depressed patients, Schutter and Van Honk [82] demonstrated that inhibitory rTMS over the left orbitofrontal cortex enhanced memory for happy faces in depressed patients, presumably by inhibiting activity in this area. The potential use of rTMS in the treatment of psychopathy remains to be studied. Potentially, rTMS could be used to enhance functioning of the orbitofrontal cortex and help to reduce impulsive tendencies. Knoch and colleagues [83] have shown that fast rTMS applied to the right dorsolateral prefrontal cortex increases activity in the orbitofrontal cortex bilaterally. As the orbitofrontal region has been associated with generating somatic markers such as anticipatory skin conductance responses to aversive stimuli, perhaps enhancing functioning of the orbitofrontal cortex could help to activate the autonomic system in psychopaths.

Finally, while psychopathic individuals tend to be resistant to treatment relative to other disorders, researchers in the field may be able to gain insight from understanding the neurobiology and biological treatments of other disorders. For example, depression has been linked to most of the same structures that have been implicated in psychopathy, but in the opposite direction. Depression has been associated with *hyper* activation in areas such as the amygdala, hippocampus, ventromedial prefrontal cortex, and anterior cingulate. As in psychopathy, it has been proposed that the connectivity between limbic and cortical areas may be disrupted, compromising the cross-talk between regions. Hyperactivity of the limbic system leads to stimulation of the hypothalamus, resulting in imbalances in the endocrine system, including increased cortisol levels [84]. Future research in psychopathy may benefit from paying attention to ongoing research on seemingly unrelated psychopathology. An exploration of the factors that may cause some individuals to develop *hyper* activity in certain brain regions while others experience *hypo* activity may provide essential clues to the development of psychopathy and other disorders. In addition, by examining the effects of various pharmacologic and behavioral treatments for disorders such as depression, we may be able to form new hypotheses about possible treatments for psychopathy.

SUMMARY

It is becoming increasingly clear that understanding the neurobiology of psychopathy goes far beyond identifying brain regions that may be involved. Genetics, neurotransmitters, and hormones all impact the functioning of brain structures and the connectivity between them. In future research it will be important to identify how these systems work together to produce the unique compilation of traits and behaviors characteristic of psychopathy. Finally, by considering the similarities and differences between psychopathy and other disorders of emotion, we may be able to gain insight into possible mechanisms that produce and maintain the disorder, as well as potential methods of treatment.

References

[1] Hare RD. Manual for the Hare psychopathy checklist-revised. Toronto: Multi-Health Systems; 1991.
[2] Skilling TA, Harris GT, Rice ME, et al. Identifying persistently antisocial offenders using the hare psychopathy checklist and DSM antisocial personality disorder criteria. Psychol Assess 2002;14(1):27–38.
[3] Hare RD. Hare psychopathy checklist–revised (PCL-R). 2nd edition. Toronto: Multi-Health Systems, Inc; 2003.
[4] Cooke DJ, Kosson DS, Michie C. Psychopathy and ethnicity: structural, item, and test generalizability of the psychopathy checklist-revised (PCL-R) in Caucasian and African American participants. Psychol Assess 2001;13:531–42.
[5] Hare RD. Psychopaths and their nature: implications for the mental health and criminal justice systems. In: Millon T, Simonsen E, Birket-Smith M, et al, editors. Psychopathy: antisocial, criminal and violent behavior. New York: Guilford Press; 1998. p. 188–212.
[6] Blair RJ, Peschardt KS, Budhani S, et al. The development of psychopathy. J Child Psychol Psychiatry 2006;47(3–4):262–76.
[7] Harris GT, Rice ME. Treatment of psychopathy: a review of empirical findings. In: Patrick CJ, editor. Handbook of pschopathy. New York: Guilford; 2006. p. 555–72.

[8] Soderstrom H, Blennow K, Manhem A, et al. CSF studies in violent offenders. I. 5-HIAA as a negative and HVA as a positive predictor of psychopathy. J Neural Transm 2001;108: 869–78.

[9] Soderstrom H, Blennow K, Sjodin A-K, et al. New evidence for an association between the CSF HVA:5-HIAA ratio and psychopathic traits. J Neurol Neurosurg Psychiatry 2003;74: 918–21.

[10] Sobczak S, Honig A, Nicolson NA, et al. Effects of acute tryptophan depletion on mood and cortisol release in first-degree relatives of type 1 and type 2 bipolar patients and healthy matched controls. Neuropsychopharmacology 2001;27(5):834–42.

[11] Porter RJ, Gallagher P, Watson S, et al. Corticosteroid-serotonin interactions in depression: a review of the human evidence. Psychopharmacology (Berl) 2004;173:1–17.

[12] Higley JD, Mehlman PT. CSF testosterone and 5-HIAA correlate with different types of aggressive behaviors. Biol Psychiatry 1996;40:1067–82.

[13] Birger M, Swartz M, Cohen D, et al. Aggression: the testosterone-serotonin link. Isr Med Assoc J 2003;5:653–8.

[14] Van Honk J, Schutter DJ. Unmasking feigned sanity: a neurobiological model of emotion processing in primary psychopathy. Cognit Neuropsychiatry 2006;11(3):285–306.

[15] Kudielka BM, Kirschbaum C. Sex differences in HPA axis responses to stress: a review. Biol Psychiatry 2005;69:113–32.

[16] Schulkin J, Gold PW, McEwen BS. Induction of corticotropin-releasing hormone gene expression by glucocorticoids: implication for understanding the states of fear and anxiety and allostatic load. Psychoneuroendocrinology 1998;23:219–43.

[17] Schulkin J. Allostasis: a neural behavioral perspective. Horm Behav 2003;43:21–7.

[18] Boissy A, Bouissou MF. Effects of androgen treatment on behavioral and physiological responses to fear-eliciting situations. Horm Behav 1994;28:66–83.

[19] Tilbrook AJ, Turner AI, Clark IJ. Effects of stress on reproduction in non-rodent mammals: the role of glucocorticoids and sex differences. Rev Reprod 2000;5:105–13.

[20] Viau V. Functional cross-talk between the hypothalamic-pituitary-gonadal and adrenal axes. J Neuroendocrinol 2002;14:506–13.

[21] Van Honk J, Peper JS, Schutter DJ. Testosterone reduces unconscious fear but not consciously experienced anxiety: implications for the disorders of fear and anxiety. Biol Psychiatry 2005;58:218–25.

[22] Van Honk J, Tuiten A, Hermans EJ, et al. A single administration of testosterone induces cardiac accelerative responses to angry faces in healthy young women. Behav Neurosci 2001;115:238–42.

[23] Van Honk J, Schutter DJ, Hermans EJ, et al. Testosterone shifts the balance between sensitivity for punishment and reward in healthy young women. Psychoneuroendocrinology 2004;29:937–43.

[24] Holi M, Auvinen-Lintunen L, Lindberg N, et al. Inverse correlation between severity of psychopathic traits and serum cortisol levels in young adult violent male offenders. Psychopathology 2006;39:102–4.

[25] Loney BR, Butler MA, Lima EN, et al. The relation between salivary cortisol, callous-unemotional traits, and conduct problems in an adolescent non-referred sample. J Child Psychol Psychiatry 2006;47(1):30–6.

[26] O'Leary MM, Loney BR, Eckel LA. Gender differences in the association between psychopathic personality traits and cortisol response to induced stress. Psychoneuroendocrinology 2006;32(2):183–91.

[27] Stalenheim EG, Eriksson E, von Knorring L, et al. Testosterone as a biological marker in psychopathy and alcoholism. Psychiatry Res 1998;77:79–88.

[28] Pajer K, Tabbah R, Gardner W, et al. Adrenal androgen and gonadal hormone levels in adolescent girls with conduct disorder. Psychoneuroendocrinology 2006;31(10): 1245–56.

[29] Maras A, Laucht M, Gerdes D, et al. Association of testosterone and dihydrotestosterone with externalizing behavior in adolescent boys and girls. Psychoneuroendocrinology 2003;28(7):932–40.
[30] Kreuz LE, Rose RM. Assessment of aggressive behavior and plasma testosterone in a young criminal population. Psychosom Med 1972;34(4):321–32.
[31] Dabbs JM, Frady RL, Carr TS. Saliva testosterone and criminal violence in young adult prison inmates. Psychosom Med 1987;49(2):174–82.
[32] Dabbs JM, Jurkovic GJ, Frady RL. Salivary testosterone and cortisol among late adolescent male offenders. J Abnorm Child Psychol 1991;19(4):469–78.
[33] Banks T, Dabbs JM. Salivary testosterone and cortisol in a delinquent and violent urban subculture. J Soc Psychol 1996;136:49–56.
[34] Mazur A, Booth A. Testosterone and dominance in men. Behav Brain Sci 1998;21:353–97.
[35] Blair RJ. Applying a cognitive neuroscience perspective to the disorder of psychopathy. Dev Psychopathol 2005;17(3):865–91.
[36] Blair RJ. Subcortical brain systems in psychopathy. In: Patrick CJ, editor. Handbook of psychopathy. New York: Guilford; 2006. p. 296–312.
[37] Flor H, Birbaumer N, Hermann C, et al. Aversive Pavlovian conditioning in psychopaths: peripheral and central correlates. Psychophysiology 2002;39:505–18.
[38] Blair RJ, Colledge E, Murray L, et al. A selective impairment in the processing of sad and fearful facial expressions in children with psychopathic tendencies. J Abnorm Child Psychol 2001;29:491–8.
[39] Newman JP, Kosson DS. Passive avoidance learning in psychopathic and nonpsychopathic offenders. J Abnorm Psychol 1986;95:252–6.
[40] Levenston GK, Patrick CJ, Bradley MM, et al. The psychopath as an observer: emotion and attention in picture processing. J Abnorm Psychol 2000;109:373–86.
[41] Blair RJ. The emergence of psychopathy: implications for the neuropsychological approach to developmental disorders. Cognition 2006;101:414–42.
[42] Yang Y, Raine A, Narr KL, et al. Amygdala volume reduction in psychopaths [abstract]. Society for Research in Psychopathology 2006.
[43] Kiehl KA, Smith AM, Hare RD, et al. Limbic abnormalities in affective processing by criminal psychopaths as revealed by functional magnetic resonance imaging. Biol Psychiatry 2001;50:677–84.
[44] Viet R, Flor H, Erb M, et al. Brain circuits involved in emotional learning in antisocial behavior and social phobia in humans. Neurosci Lett 2002;328:233–6.
[45] Birbaumer N, Viet R, Lotze M, et al. Deficient fear conditioning in psychopathy: a functional magnetic resonance imaging study. Arch Gen Psychiatry 2005;62(7):799–805.
[46] Rilling JK, Glenn AL, Jairam MR, et al. Neural correlates of social cooperation and non-cooperation as a function of psychopathy. Biol Psychiatry 2007;61:1260–71.
[47] Gordon H. Functional differences among those high and low on a trait measure of psychopathy. Biol Psychiatry 2004;56:516–21.
[48] Muller JL, Sommer M, Wagner V, et al. Abnormalities in emotion processing within cortical and subcortical regions in criminal psychopaths: evidence from a functional magnetic resonance imaging study using pictures with emotional content. Psychiatry Res 2003;54:152–62.
[49] Schneider F, Habel U, Kessler C, et al. Functional imaging of conditioned aversive emotional responses in antisocial personality disorder. Neuropsychobiology 2000;42:192–201.
[50] Blair RJ. The amygdala and ventromedial prefrontal cortex in morality and psychopathy. Trends Cogn Sci 2007;11(9):387–92.
[51] Brown SM, Hariri AR. Neuroimaging studies of serotonin gene polymorphisms: exploring the interplay of genes, brain, and behavior. Cogn Affect Behav Neurosci 2006;6:44–52.

[52] Finger EC, Marsh AA, Buzas B, et al. The impact of tryptophan depletion and 5-HTTLPR genotype on passive avoidance and response reversal instrumental learning tasks. Neuropsychopharmacology 2007;32(1):206–15.

[53] Raine A, Ishikawa SS, Arce E, et al. Hippocampal structural asymmetry in unsuccessful psychopaths. Biol Psychiatry 2004;55:185–91.

[54] Best CT. The emergence of cerebral asymmetries in early human development: a literature review and a neuroembryological model. In: Molfese DL, Segalowitz SJ, editors. Brain lateralization in children: developmental implications. New York: Guilford Press; 1988. p. 5–34.

[55] Szabo CA, Wyllie E, Siavalas EL, et al. Hippocampal volumetry in children 6 years or younger: assessment of children with and without complex febrile seizures. Epilepsy Res 1999;33:1–9.

[56] Laakso MP, Vaurio O, Koivisto E, et al. Psychopathy and the posterior hippocampus. Behav Brain Res 2001;118:187–93.

[57] Raine A, Lencz T, Bihrle S, et al. Reduced prefrontal gray matter volume and reduced autonomic activity in antisocial personality disorder. Arch Gen Psychiatry 2000;57:119–27.

[58] Van Honk J, Schutter DJ, d'Alfonso AAL, et al. Repetitive transcranial magnetic stimulation at the frontopolar cortex reduces skin conductance but not heart rate: reduced gray matter excitability in orbitofrontal regions. Arch Gen Psychiatry 2001;58:973–4.

[59] Yang Y, Raine A, Lencz T, et al. Volume reduction in prefrontal gray matter in unsuccessful criminal psychopaths. Biol Psychiatry 2005;15(57):1103–8.

[60] Laakso MP, Gunning-Dixon F, Vaurio O, et al. Prefrontal volumes in habitually violent subjects with antisocial personality disorder and type 2 alcoholism. Psychiatry Res 2002;114:95–102.

[61] Yang Y, Raine A, Narr KL, et al. Successful and unsuccessful psychopaths: neuroanatomical similarities and differences [abstract]. Hum Brain Mapp 2006.

[62] Rilling JK, Gutman DA, Zeh TR, et al. A neural basis for social cooperation. Neuron 2002;35(2):395–405.

[63] Mitchell DG, Colledge E, Leonard A, et al. Risky decisions and response reversal: is there evidence of orbitofrontal cortex dysfunction in psychopathic individuals? Neuropsychologia 2002;40(12):2013–22.

[64] Anderson SW, Bechara A, Damasio H, et al. Impairment of social and moral behavior related to early damage in human prefrontal cortex. Nat Neurosci 1999;2:1031–7.

[65] Intrator J, Hare RD, Stritzke P, et al. A brain imaging (single photon emission computerized tomography) study of semantic and affective processing in psychopaths. Biol Psychiatry 1997;42:96–103.

[66] Kiehl KA, Smith AM, Mendrek A, et al. Temporal lobe abnormalities in semantic processing by criminal psychopaths as revealed by functional magnetic resonance imaging. Psychiatry Res 2004;130:27–42.

[67] Critchley HD, Mathias CJ, Dolan RJ, et al. Fear conditioning in humans: the influence of awareness and autonomic arousal on functional neuroanatomy. Neuron 2002;33:653–63.

[68] Kiehl KA. A cognitive neuroscience perspective on psychopathy: evidence for paralimbic system dysfunction. Psychiatry Res 2006;142:107–28.

[69] Damasio AR. Descartes' error: emotion, reason, and the human brain. New York: GP Putnam's Sons; 1994.

[70] Bechara A, Damasio H, Damasio AR, et al. Role of the amygdala in decision-making. Ann N Y Acad Sci 2003;985:356–69.

[71] Buckholtz JW, Callicott JH, Kolachana B, et al. Genetic variation in MAOA modulates ventromedial prefrontal circuitry mediating individual differences in human personality. Mol Psychiatry 2008;13:313–24.

[72] Davidson RJ, Putnam KM, Larson CL. Dysfunction in the neural circuitry of emotion regulation—a possible prelude to violence. Science 2000;289:591–4.

[73] Schutter DJ, Van Honk J. Salivary cortisol levels and the coupling of midfrontal delta-beta oscillations. Int J Psychophysiol 2005;55(1):127–9.

[74] Schutter DJ, Van Honk J. Decoupling of midfrontal delta-beta oscillations after testosterone administration. Int J Psychophysiol 2004;53(1):71–3.

[75] Hiatt KD, Newman JP. Behavioral evidence of prolonged interhemispheric transfer time among psychopathic offenders. Neuropsychology 2007;21(3):313–8.

[76] Raine A, Lencz T, Taylor K, et al. Corpus callosum abnormalities in psychopathic antisocial individuals. Arch Gen Psychiatry 2003;60:1134–42.

[77] Glenn AL, Raine A, Venables PH, et al. Early temperamental and psychophysiological precursors of adult psychopathic personality. J Abnorm Psychol 2007;116(3):508–18.

[78] Frick PJ, O'Brien BS, Wooton JM, et al. Psychopathy and conduct problems in children. J Abnorm Psychol 1994;103(4):700–7.

[79] Loney BR, Frick PJ, Clements CB, et al. Emotional reactivity and callous unemotional traits in adolescents. J Clin Child Adolesc Psychol 2003;32(1):66–80.

[80] Burt T, Lisanby SH, Sackeim HA. Neuropsychiatric applications of transcranial magnetic stimulation: a meta analysis. Int J Neuropsychopharmacol 2002;5:73–103.

[81] Mayberg HS, Liotti M, Brannan SK, et al. Reciprocal limbic-cortical function and negative mood: converging PET findings in depression and normal sadness. Am J Psychiatry 1999;156:675–82.

[82] Schutter DJ, Van Honk J. Increased positive emotional memory after repetitive transcranial magnetic stimulation over the orbitofrontal cortex. J Psychiatry Neurosci 2006;31(2):101–4.

[83] Knoch D, Treyer V, Regard M, et al. Lateralized and frequency-dependent effects of prefrontal rTMS on regional cerebral blood flow. NeuroImage 2006;31(2):641–8.

[84] Maletic V, Robinson M, Oakes T, et al. Neurobiology of depression: an integrated view of key findings. Int J Clin Pract 2007;61(12):2030–40.

Child Development and Personality Disorder

Patricia Cohen, PhD

Columbia University College of Physicians & Surgeons and New York State
Psychiatric Institute, 1051 Riverside Drive, New York, NY 10032, USA

Empirical data on personality disorder in childhood and adolescence have been sparse until the past decade. There are several probable reasons for this, including the separation of "disorders beginning in childhood" as a category in the Diagnostic and Statistical Manual of Mental Disorders (DSM) [1], and the assumption by the DSM of instability of personality in childhood ("It should be recognized that the traits of a Personality Disorder that appear in childhood will often not persist unchanged into adult life."). The DSM was not wrong on this issue: behavior and personality patterns are less stable in childhood and adolescence; however, it is increasingly realized that this is a matter of degree of stability compared with adults. Longitudinal studies of carefully diagnosed patients [2,3] have shown that variation over time in personality disorder (PD) symptom pattern and level in adulthood is also typical.

Two other gradual changes in empirically founded theoretical perspectives have also contributed to the beginning of a blossoming in empirical work relevant to the development of personality disorder. One is the increasing appreciation that most mental disorders have prodromal signs or even onset much earlier in life than is implicit in an adult-oriented diagnostic system. For example, the National Comorbidity Survey Replication found half of all lifetime cases of anxiety, mood, impulse-control, and substance use disorders to have started by age 14 by retrospective report [4]. Another reason for a growth in interest in developmental issues in PD is the increasing appreciation of the complexity of gene and environmental causes of all mental disorders reflected in empirical work based on human and animal models [5]. But ideal developmental studies begin early in life, are longitudinal, and include a wide range of prospectively collected potential risks and precursors of the disorders being studied. Some studies may be based on children with diagnosable or clear PD spectrum symptomatic elevation. Other studies may be based on a large enough general population to include a number of likely PD-vulnerable

E-mail address: cohenpa@pi.cpmc.columbia.edu

0193-953X/08/$ – see front matter
doi:10.1016/j.psc.2008.03.005

children. Such studies, of course, must be performed in real time, and thus require investigator commitment and funding over an extended period.

To date, the only long-term PD study beginning in early childhood and assessing PD by early adolescence is the Children in the Community (CIC) study of a randomly selected cohort of about 800 American children first studied at a mean age of 6 and first assessed for all Axis I and Axis II mental disorders at mean age of 13.5 [6]. The cohort will be about mean age 38 on completion of the current assessment of all mental disorders in 2009.

An earlier review on vulnerability to personality disorder [7] noted the sparseness of prospectively measured (or even retrospective) data on childhood characteristics preceding PD. In consequence, they focused on seven kinds of PD symptoms that are diagnostic criteria for one or more PDs: (1) a hostile, paranoid world view; (2) intense, unstable, inappropriate, or flat emotion; (3) impulsivity or rigidity; (4) overly close or distant/avoidant relationships; (5) extreme or absent sense of self; (6) peculiar thought processes and behaviors; and (7) psychopathy. Each of these symptom sets has at least some relevant research history in the area of child development, although generally no direct evidence of prediction of later PD.

WHAT IS "PERSONALITY" AND HOW DOES IT DEVELOP?

Actual empirical studies of the development of PD covering more than a limited section of the period from birth or very early life to adulthood are sparse. Nevertheless, the last decade has been a very fertile one for increasing convergence on models of personality development, arising in particular from evolving conceptions of the origins and role of personality. These newer models present personality as arising from the combination of basic and universal emotions and emotion-related experience. A recent integration of this emerging consensus is provided by Izard [8], who calls upon a broad literature from biological and brain studies to animal models. Izard [8] views emotions as the source of "universal capacities to regulate and motivate cognition and action independent of the cyclic processes that characterize homeostasis and physiological drive states." Six emotions are considered to be basic because they are unlearned and universal (although varying in strength across individuals) and "preempt consciousness." These are interest, joy/happiness, sadness, anger, disgust, and fear. Interest and joy/happiness are functional at birth and the others are functional within the first 2 years. As Jack Block [9] has indicated in the title of his book, Personality as an Affect-Regulating System this theoretical stance is also consistent with his general perspective, although Block views the most fundamental affect as anxiety produced by perceived or experienced danger, beginning in early childhood.

A two-dimensional view of children's problems reflected in Block's relatively simple classification of children into undercontrolled, overcontrolled, and resilient (the low-problem group) also matches the basic dimensions also found in measures of parental descriptions of the emotional/behavioral problems of young offspring. Thus, Achenbach's Child Behavior Check

List (CBCL) [10] descriptions of problematic child behavior show a clear (if higher-order) two- (correlated) factor structure, internalizing (including elements reflecting overcontrol) and externalizing (undercontrol) problems. However, more recent analyses of CBCL dimensions as assessed in general rather than clinical populations indicate that even when the data are limited to a problem checklist a more discriminating series of eight factors or dimensions are also measurable. The identified dimensions of problems as reflected in the CBCL administered in unselected adolescent populations as well as clinical samples in 30 different countries include anxious/depressed, withdrawn/depressed, somatic complaints, social problems, thought problems, attention problems, rule-breaking behavior, and aggression [11]. Furthermore, these dimensions are closely matched by those based on adult self-report of the same problems [12].

Over time, the basic positive and negative emotions are gradually replaced by emotion schemas in which cognitive frames, appraisals, and attributions develop out of the individual's emotional experience and replace the basic emotions as the predominant motivators. These "motivators" may be seen as temperament in early childhood, in a period in which it may be normative that biological differences may have a dominant influence. With increasing age, the schemas combine these emotional states in relatively common/correlated patterns but more-or-less uniquely across individuals, based on genetic and experiential combinations. Thus, personality differences develop from combinations of individual genetic-based differences in the relative strength of these emotions and life experiences that shape the nature of the individual's schema regarding self, others, and the world they live in. The development of personality over the next decades takes place as a series of adaptations to subsequent threats and pleasures, shaped by the individual's biological heritage, by the exposures experienced, and by the individual's emerging/changing interpretation of the world. Gradually, "stable coherent families of emotional schemas may become organized as personality traits" [8]. The relatively high heritabilities of personality disorder features from early childhood have been demonstrated in a young twin sample [13]. Caspi and colleagues [14] present an excellent fusion of the literature on the development of personality from early childhood throughout life and Shiner [15] applies this literature specifically to personality disorder.

Early Temperament Differences as Potential Precursors of Later Personality Disorder

Early temperament as reflected in Rothbart's Children's Behavior Questionnaire [16] reflects the Izard emotional dimensions in large part, including anger, fear and shyness, smiling/laughter/pleasure/approach, and attention focusing and inhibitory control, covering the overall variation in affective, activation, and attentional aspects of personality. Thus, this literature is potentially relevant to understanding early aspects of the constructive and disordered development of personality.

In a factor analysis of maternal reports of age 2 to 10 offspring, Cohen [17] found seven dimensions of mother-reported temperament variation and problems including anger, activity level, persistence, impulsivity, demanding, fearful, and negative mood in the CIC representative general population sample. Second-order factors combined anger, impulsivity, nonpersistence, and high activity in the first "difficult" factor and fearful, demanding, and negative mood in the second (inhibited). These dimensions resemble those identified by Thomas and Chess [18], and indeed the original items were based on their work. These higher-order "temperament" factors are also relatively consistent with those identified by Digman [19] whose data on school-age children were the source of the "big five" movement.

A grouping of these same temperament reports into those reflecting behavior problems, depressive problems, anxiety/fear, and immaturity at mean age 8 were used to predict persistent disorder in each of the three PD clusters assessed twice in adolescence [20]. Behavior problems predicted disorders in all three clusters with elevated odds of about 20% to 30% above average for those with such problems 1 SD above the mean. Depressive problems predicted Clusters A and B, each with odds about 40% higher for each SD. The anxiety problems, somewhat surprisingly, significantly predicted only Cluster B (with Odds Ratio = 1.23), whereas immaturity predicted all three clusters at about 20% to 30% higher rates for each SD increase. Sex differences were also present, among which the most interesting may be the prediction of persistent Cluster A disorder by behavior problems only in girls, and by depressive symptoms only in boys in analyses in which all early problem sets were included as predictors. New analyses of early temperament and personality disorder stability from adolescence to mid-adulthood of this cohort have not as yet been reported.

ASSESSMENT OF PERSONALITY DISORDER OR COMPONENTS OF PERSONALITY DISORDER IN CHILDHOOD: CURRENT STATUS

An examination of the published empirical literature on developmental aspects of PD shows that most of this work focuses either on borderline or antisocial PD.

Antisocial Personality Disorder

The literature relevant to early precursors of antisocial PD is substantial because it falls into the separate research domains of criminology and psychiatric disability [21,22]. Nevertheless, the connection between these two professional perspectives when focused on childhood is surprisingly tenuous, especially in view of the high fraction of childhood cases in clinical mental health services whose essential problems as viewed by parents and/or teachers are in the realm of antisocial behavior. And childhood assessments tend to be framed by the definitions of the diagnostic system including opposition/defiant (ODD) and conduct disorder (CD), which focus on behaviors rather than potentially underlying personality components that may motivate such behaviors and predict the discriminating aspects of adult antisocial PD. Some part of this professional perspective may be a reflection of awareness that these disorders and elevated symptoms of these disorders are often time-limited in adolescence, and perhaps even a (dissocial) indicator of a maturational process. No effort will be made here to summarize the voluminous literature on the course and prediction into adulthood of these disorders; however, it is worth reviewing the personality component of adult antisocial disorder as viewed by criminologists, and the efforts to assess this prospectively in childhood.

Perhaps the most researched of the constructs that assess a central "personality" component of an adult PD is low empathy/callousness-unemotionality in children as precursors of antisocial PD. Farrington [23] presents a plea for assessment of childhood psychopathy, based on current evidence regarding its long-term importance [22,24]. Several measures of this construct are available, including the Basic Empathy Scale [25]. A clinically intended measure developed from items in Millon's Adolescent Clinical Inventory was shown to have predictive validity [26]. Evidence of a taxonic structure of psychopathy in youth that is independent of a broader antisocial behavior taxon has been reported [27]. Thus longitudinal evidence of the influence of early problems in this domain on more stable psychopathy and subsequent antisocial personality disorder is accumulating [22,28]; nevertheless, it is not clear that adoption of any of the several available measures is widespread in clinical settings.

Broader measures of deficiencies in understanding the perspectives and problems of others, including other children, are under development and experimental use [29,30]. The theoretical link between difficulties or delay of this basic interpersonal understanding and problems in subsequent social behavior, a central component of all personality disorders, would appear to be strong [31,32]. Thus, a potential future research extension of this aspect of early personality development risk may include issues of the developmental timing of "theory of mind" in infants and toddlers.

With regard to childhood development preceding adult antisocial PD, a recent concise summary of the eight leading theories of the development of chronic adult criminality is available in Farrington [33].

Borderline Personality Disorder

The Borderline Personality Features Scale [34] has been shown to be moderately stable over 1 year as self-reported by fourth- to sixth-grade children. School-aged children with and without a history of maltreatment have been shown to differ on a composite measure of borderline PD precursors [35].

Previously, the clinical diagnosis of borderline disorder in childhood or early adolescence has often been made upon presentation of a patient with a broad mix of problems including both "internalizing" symptoms such as anxiety and depression and "externalizing" symptoms such as impulsivity, defiance and oppositional behavior, and potential psychotic experiences and antisocial and/or substance abuse problems. Such patients typically also show suicidal or parasuicidal behavior, problems in relationships with family and peers, and extreme dysfunction. This diagnosis often represents a mixed set of problems implying very poor prognosis that do not necessarily meet DSM borderline disorder criteria for adults. And, indeed, the follow-up studies thus far do not suggest that a large fraction of these children or adolescents will meet criteria for borderline disorder as adults, although they will not generally "recover" to function in the normative range either. It is possible that the general clinical diagnosis of borderline disorder in seriously dysfunctional patients at any age may have been a contributor to the very negative view of this disorder by professionals in the field and a reluctance to diagnose this or any other personality disorder in children or adolescents. Thus, although measures of borderline disorder can be reliably assessed in adolescents [36], its discriminant validity in patient samples may be problematic [37]. Nevertheless, a few clinical studies of childhood borderline disorder meeting DSM-III-R or -IV criteria are beginning to be available. Using a clinical sample of school-aged children, Zelkowitz and colleagues [38] found that children meeting criteria for borderline pathology also showed deficits in executive function, which predicted borderline pathology independently of trauma history.

ASSESSMENT OF PERSONALITY DISORDER IN CHILDREN AND ADOLESCENTS

Several measures of most or all PD disorders or symptoms in children or adolescents have been developed and employed. The Schedler-Westen Assessment Procedure-200 for Adolescents [39] is a Q-sort instrument designed for clinicians to use for adolescent patients. An assessment based on a checklist of the DSM criteria has also been shown to relate to other variables comparably to a structured diagnostic interview and thus provides a reasonable substitute. In addition, this research team obtained a global clinical rating of the extent to which the adolescent resembled each PD as described in the text of DSM-IV. These ratings showed good correlations with the criterion sum for the same disorder and more modest correlations with criteria of other PDs [40]. Some caution may appropriately accompany these methods because the study sample on which they were employed was selected by a national sample of clinicians as the last adolescent patient they had seen "whose personality they felt they knew." A summary review of adolescent personality pathology assessment by this research team is also available [39].

The Coolidge Personality and Neuropsychosocial Inventory for Children [41] is a parent report instrument designed to assess all PDs in offspring between the ages of 5 and 17. It has been employed in a sample of 112 twin pairs at mean age 8.7 years to estimate heritabilities [13]. Larger monozygotic than dizygotic twin correlations for all PDs except passive-aggressive were shown, with the greatest ratio for conduct disorder (used as a childhood substitute for antisocial PD).

The CIC study originally adapted items from the Personality Disorder Questionnaire (PDQ) self-report adult measure [42] and adopted or wrote other items to replace age-inappropriate items [6]. The particular items selected from this large protocol for these measures underwent several changes as the DSM-III changed to -III-R to -IV; as the cohort reached full adulthood necessarily self-report replaced combined self- and parent report, and clinical assessments were added [43]. Analyses of CIC data over the past few years have strongly suggested that when the goal is discriminating among the members of a general population sample, self-report may be about as adequate a reflection of PD symptoms as combined self-mother report even in early adolescence. Adaptations of the study's self-report measures have been developed and employed in several new studies with apparently good utility of responses [44].

A fairly comprehensive coverage of PD symptoms in childhood is reflected in the scales of the Dimensional Personality Symptom Items, which was modeled on Livesley's Dimensional Assessment of Personality Pathology designed for adults [45].

PROSPECTIVELY OR CURRENTLY ASSESSED CHILDHOOD RISKS FOR PERSONALITY DISORDER

Demographic Risks for Pre-Adult Personality Disorder

Analyses undertaken for somewhat different purposes showed a series of risks reported in early childhood to predict an aggregate measure of PD symptoms in both late adolescence and early adulthood. These risks include low socioeconomic status (SES) of family, being raised in a single-parent family, welfare support of family, parental death, and social isolation [46]. In aggregate, the early adolescent risks predicted 28% of the variance in PD symptoms 9 years later in adulthood. Related analyses looking at early risks for PD disorders by cluster demonstrated these SES effects over the same period [47]. A more recent study of the 2-decade course of borderline and schizotypal symptoms to cohort mean age 33 indicated an unabated and independent association of low family of origin (FO) SES with elevated symptoms of both disorders, net of potentially correlated effects of IQ, history of abuse, and problematic parenting [48]. Such findings suggest the environment and status of the family have strong and lasting effects on the social schemas that develop around the basic emotions and associated brain functions. In fact, these associations are so universal that FO SES is included as a "control" variable in virtually every analysis based on the CIC data. Excess parental divorce, substance abuse, and criminality were also reported in a young child clinical sample with borderline disorder in comparison with those without borderline disorder [49].

Physical Health Problems

Prenatal exposure to the Dutch famine in the WWII period has been shown to predict subsequent antisocial PD [50]. Pre- or perinatal problems may also result in lower intellectual function, which tends to be a (modest) risk for PD in adolescence and adulthood [46], particularly for symptoms of borderline and schizotypal PD [48]. In analyses not yet published, health problems in the infant's first year showed a modest but significant relationship with any PD assessed at mean age 13 by combined mother and child report in the CIC study.

Early Attachment Problems

A theoretically powerful early childhood risk for subsequent personality disorder is problematic attachment to parents, especially to mother. Attachment theory views early developmental experience as leading to a working model of the world, and particularly of reasonable expectations of social interaction [51]. These experiences seem particularly relevant to the development of PD because of the central component of social schema in PD and the expectation that such working models may be self-perpetuating by the behavioral responses that they tend to evoke. Attachment theory arose from Bowlby's [52] early focus on the infant's motivation for exploration and mastery, and the need for a secure base of operation. Despite probable differences in perspectives among child development researchers, this theory and the empirical evidence would seem to fit fairly well with Izard's [8] view of the factors that shape personality. Recent empirical tests of the relationships between PDs and attachment in adolescents and adults have been performed but no infants with different measured attachment patterns have been studied longitudinally with regard to personality disorder in late childhood, adolescence, or adulthood.

The alternative methods of assessing attachment in adolescents and adults remain a controversial topic that has been well reviewed [40]. Clinicians' ratings on the match between an adolescent patient and prototypes of secure, dismissive, preoccupied, and disorganized attachment were correlated with ratings of match with PDs. All PD ratings were negatively correlated with secure attachment, except histrionic, dependent, and obsessive PD. All cluster A PDs and avoidant PD were related to dismissing attachment, borderline, and dependent PD with preoccupied attachment, and cluster A PDs and borderline disorder with disorganized attachment. A study of clinical ratings of adult patients showed a similar correlational pattern.

Although attachment itself was not assessed in a comparison of 7- to 12-year-old children with borderline and nonborderline disorders in a day treatment program, those with borderline disorders had higher rates of foster placement (22% versus 13%) and parental divorce (80.5% versus 50.9%) [49].

Self-report measures of anxious and avoidant attachment in mid-adolescence were used to assess the independent prediction of PDs in the three diagnostic clusters in the emerging adulthood period and about a decade later at mean age 33 [53]. Interpersonal aggression was also employed as a control: high anxious attachment consistently predicted both Cluster B and Cluster C symptoms, whereas high avoidant attachment consistently predicted Cluster A symptoms and was consistently negatively related to Cluster C symptoms.

Parenting and Parent-Child Relationship

In the first report of risk for PD in a general population of adolescents (the CIC sample), Bezirganian and colleagues [54] reported that earlier maternal inconsistency with overinvolvement predicted both new-onset and persistent borderline disorder in adolescent offspring. The evidence of a PD predictive role for problematic parenting, and especially power assertive or harsh punishment and low affection is accumulating in prospective data [55]. In this study, either or both aspects of problematic parenting assessed in adolescence predicted each Cluster A disorder; antisocial and borderline PD; and avoidant, passive-aggressive, and depressive PD in adulthood.

CHILDHOOD ABUSE AND NEGLECT AS PREDICTORS OF PERSONALITY DISORDER

A recent literature review has provided a detailed summary of published research findings regarding the empirically demonstrated associations of childhood physical, sexual, and emotional abuse, and childhood neglect with PD during adolescence or adulthood [56]. These different forms of abuse or neglect often occur together and reflect general severely inadequate or even malevolent parenting, but sexual abuse in particular may often not involve parents except as inadequate supervisors and protectors of offspring. Because they may have different implications for our understanding of their shaping influence on personality development, we note here where a given kind of childhood abuse or neglect appears to have effects on PD development that is independent of other kinds on the basis of at least one study.

Childhood physical abuse predicts antisocial, borderline, and schizotypal PD, independent of the effects of other types of childhood maltreatment; depressive, paranoid, passive-aggressive, and schizoid PD traits are also elevated following physical abuse but not independently of other abuse. Sexual abuse predicts every PD and PD symptom measure (traits) except dependent PD, and predicts borderline PD and histrionic and depressive PD traits net of other kinds of maltreatment. Childhood emotional abuse predicts borderline PD independent of other types of childhood maltreatment, as well as avoidant, depressive, narcissistic, obsessive-compulsive, paranoid, schizoid, and schizotypal PD traits.

Childhood neglect predicts subsequent avoidant, borderline, passive-aggressive, antisocial, and schizotypal PDs, independently of the effects of other types of child maltreatment, as well as dependent, narcissistic, paranoid, and schizoid PD traits. Further work on specific kinds of childhood neglect suggest that physical neglect may be differentially associated with traits of specific PDs. Despite these correlations, it is also clear that the child's perception of the meaning of the experience is an important element of its ultimate effect [57].

In clinical cases of childhood borderline disorder, sexual abuse and severe neglect were each higher in the history of these children in comparison with young children without borderline disorder in the same day treatment program [49]. This finding confirmed parallel findings reported earlier on the basis of clinical chart review [58].

OTHER SPECIFIC EARLY SIGNS OF PERSONALITY DISORDER

Although data on neurobiological correlates of childhood PD is yet to be widely explored, two indicators of problematic executive function, the Wisconsin Card Sorting Test and the Continuous Performance Test have been shown to be abnormal in school-age day treatment children with borderline pathology [59].

Early social inhibition has been shown to be associated with avoidant disorder in young offspring of parents with panic disorder, major depression, both, and neither [60]. Self-mutilation in childhood has been self-reported by adult patients with borderline disorder [61]. Other suicidal threats or behavior are also part of the history reported by adult borderline patients or their families, although unambiguous prospectively assessed suicidal behavior in childhood is thus far absent. Axis I disorders as comorbid, developmentally earlier, or subsequent are discussed later in this article. In the CIC study [62,63], adolescents with prosocial life goals were more likely to show a decline in PD as they moved into adulthood than were those with more materialistic and self-oriented goals.

Efforts to frame early temperament, personality, and developmental psychopathology in ways that facilitate the assessment of childhood risks and early manifestations of personality disorder are under way [64,65].

STABILITY OF PERSONALITY DISORDER FROM CHILDHOOD TO ADULTHOOD

Chronicity of adult personality disorder is associated with early onset as retrospectively reported in clinical populations [66]. Early adolescent clinical cases of disruptive behavior disorders were more likely to have Cluster B disorders at mean age 43, and adolescent girls with emotional disorders had elevated rates of Cluster C PD [67]. Nevertheless, early symptoms of PD are not necessarily followed by adult disorder. Most of the current data on the course of personality disorder in childhood and early adulthood comes from longitudinal studies of nonpatient population samples. Regardless of the method of assessment (combined parent and child, self-report only, and DSM-III-R or DSM-IV-based), symptoms of each PD and thus the prevalence of each PD declines with age, at least from age 9 through the mid-twenties [43,68–70]. In the CIC study, where these assessments began as early as age 9, it is likely that some of this decline is related to simple developmental maturation with regard to social skills and appreciation of cultural expectations by both peers and adults (eg, with respect to histrionic and narcissistic behavior) [69]. Disorders show somewhat more stability over time than certain Axis I disorders, such as major depressive disorder (which is episodic by definition) and childhood behavior disorders such as ODD and CD (which are generally not diagnosed in adulthood), but a full comparison of continuity over time among the PDs and between PDs and Axis I disorders has not as yet been performed in either clinical or general population samples. Adolescent PD not otherwise specified (NOS) was associated with increases of 3 to 4 times the odds of adult Cluster A, B, and C disorders 6 years later in young adulthood [71].

PREDICTIVE RELATIONSHIPS AND COMORBIDITY OF CHILDHOOD/ADOLESCENT AXIS I DISORDERS AND PERSONALITY DISORDERS

Comorbidity among the PDs in adolescence was high in the CIC cohort, with about half of those with any PD also meeting diagnostic criteria for one or more other PDs [69]. An effort to understand this relationship was examined in a study of potential reciprocal effects of longitudinal courses of borderline and narcissistic PD symptoms from adolescence to adulthood [72]. Both sets of symptoms are highest in the early adolescent period, and correlated throughout. When narcissistic PD symptoms are high relative to borderline symptoms in early adolescence, both sets of symptoms tend to decline substantially, interpreted by the authors as a benign developmental delay subsequently compensated. In contrast, when borderline PD symptoms were high relative to narcissistic symptoms, the period following was characterized by a rise in narcissistic symptoms, viewed as a developmental "process gone awry" [72].

In clinical samples of adolescent and adult hospitalized patients with borderline disorder comorbidity with other PDs was shown to be higher in adolescence than in the adults [73], again potentially attributable to the immaturity reflected in symptoms of most or all PDs.

Comorbidity between early adolescent PDs and Axis I disorders is also very substantial, with about half of the early adolescents who had a disorder in one Axis likely to also have a disorder in the other in the CIC epidemiologic sample [74]. Such high comorbidity has also been shown in the few recent studies of PD in clinical samples of children. In their clinical sample of young boys with borderline disorder, Guzder and colleagues [49] found 25 (81%) of 31 had comorbid conduct disorder. In the full sample of girls and boys with borderline disorder, 67.5% also met criteria for ADHD, 47.5% for ODD, 22.5% for major depression, and 30% for overanxious disorder.

Both Axis I emotional and behavioral disorders in adolescence predict adult PDs [67], although the absence of earlier assessment in this study leaves open the questions of potential existence of these PDs in adolescence and reciprocal prediction across Axes. In the CIC study, the number of early adolescent Axis I disorders also predicted adult PDs 9 years later, to a maximum of 56% of those with four or more Axis I disorders having an adult Cluster A PD, 50% having a Cluster B PD, and 38% having a Cluster C PD [75]. These high prevalences contrast with prevalences of 4%, 12%, and 4% in those with no earlier Axis I disorder. The odds of schizoid, narcissistic, and antisocial PD in young adulthood increased by about five to six times among youth with a disruptive disorder in adolescence and the odds of adult paranoid PD increased about four times among adolescents with an anxiety disorder [76]. Early major depressive disorder (MDD) predicted both Cluster B and Cluster C PDs [75] and was a powerful predictor of adult antisocial PD [76]. Panic attacks in early adolescence also predict adult PD in each of the PD clusters [77].

Borderline, dependent, depressive, histrionic, and schizotypal symptom means over adolescence predicted MDD or dysthymic disorder over a decade later net of comorbid Axis I disorders in adolescence [78]. Early adolescent PD and CD were predictors of subsequent symptoms and diagnoses of substance abuse or dependence independently of other Axis I disorders and family risks. Analyses over 20 years indicated Cluster B disorder to be independent risks for new-onset substance use disorder (SUD) [79]. Early adolescent Axis I and Axis

II comorbidity showed the strongest prediction of treatment for mental illness including psychotropic drug use 20 years later [80]. Some measures of mid-adulthood disorder and dysfunction were more associated with Axis I disorder without PD 20 years earlier, and others more associated with PD without Axis I disorder 20 years earlier. However, almost all such measures were most negatively affected by early across-Axis comorbidity often essentially approximating an additive effect [74]. The high level of comorbidity suggests that much negative prognosis currently attributed to Axis I disorders may be attributable to these disorders.

PROGNOSTIC IMPLICATIONS OF EARLY PERSONALITY DISORDER AND ELEVATED PERSONALITY DISORDER SYMPTOMS

Findings are beginning to accumulate regarding the long-term functional prognosis associated with PD assessed in adolescence. Several studies of the CIC cohort investigated prognostic implications of adolescent PD for young adult problems (mean age 22). Crawford and colleagues [81] showed a prediction by adolescent Cluster B PD of low intimacy and well-being that increased as young people entered adulthood. Conflict with family members was high during the transition to adulthood (ages 17 to 27) for those with earlier paranoid, schizotypal, and narcissistic PD, and except for paranoid PD these effects were independent of comorbid Axis I disorders [82]. Both Axis I disorders and adolescent PDs predicted more negative young adult quality of life, with the most negative outcomes generally attributable to across-Axis comorbidity [83]. Over this same period, Cluster A symptoms in adolescence were associated with early parenthood and less advanced education (net of controls), the former in sharp contrast with expectations based on ultimate lower fertility in persons with full schizophrenia [84]. Ehrensaft and colleagues [85] showed continuity of PD symptoms from adolescence into early adulthood predicted subsequent partner violence and Johnson and colleagues [86] showed that the risk of violence in those with a PD history was twice as large as in those without such a history, with both Clusters A and B predicting significantly.

Adolescents with PD in each of the three diagnostic clusters showed substantially lower quality of life (QOL) in adulthood in the fourth decade of life [87]. Highest negative effects were for those with disorders in Cluster B; nevertheless, the effects of each of the PD clusters showed independent associations. Effects of adolescent borderline and schizotypal PD symptoms showed QOL reductions independent of comorbid disorders. Analyses of adolescents with borderline disorder or high symptoms in the CIC study are in press, showing functional problems over the following 20 years [88] including effects independent of early major depressive disorder or conduct disorder.

In sum, based on the CIC study, the evidence is surprisingly strong that even early adolescent personality disorders or elevated personality disorder symptoms have a broad range of negative effects well into adulthood, for the most part comparable to or even larger than those of Axis I disorders. Current evidence suggests that the most severe long-term prognosis is associated with borderline and schizotypal PDs and elevated symptoms. And, of course, childhood conduct disorder is in a peculiar status, disappearing in adulthood to be manifest as a very severe disorder—antisocial PD—in a minority of those with the adolescent disorder.

References

[1] American Psychiatric Association. Diagnostic and statistical manual of mental disorders. 4th edition. Washington, DC: Author; 1994. p. 631.

[2] McGlashan TH, Grilo CM, Sanislow CA, et al. Two-year prevalence and stability of individual DSM-IV criteria for schizotypal, borderline, avoidant, and obsessive-compulsive personality disorders: toward a hybrid model of axis II disorders. Am J Psychiatry 2005;162(5): 883–9.

[3] Zanarini MC, Frankenburg FR, Hennen J, et al. The longitudinal course of borderline psychopathology: 6-year prospective follow-up of the phenomenology of borderline personality disorder. Am J Psychiatry 2003;160(2):274–83.

[4] Kessler RC, Berglund P, Demler O, et al. Lifetime prevalence and age-of-onset distributions of DSM-IV disorders in the national comorbidity survey replication. Arch Gen Psychiatry 2005;62(6):593–602.

[5] Penke L, Denissen JA, Miller GF. The evolutionary genetics of personality. European Journal of Personality 2007;21(5):549–87.

[6] Cohen P, Crawford T. Developmental issues. In: Oldham JM, Skodol AE, Bender DS, editors. The American Psychiatric Publishing textbook of personality disorders. Washington, DC: American Psychiatric Publishing, Inc.; 2005. p. 171–85.

[7] Geiger TC, Crick NR. A developmental psychopathology perspective on vulnerability to personality disorders. In: Ingram RE, Price JM, editors. Vulnerability to psychopathology: risk across the lifespan. New York: Guilford Press; 2001. p. 57–102.

[8] Izard CE. Basic emotions, natural kinds, emotion schemas, and a new paradigm. Perspectives on Psychological Science 2007;2(3):260–80.

[9] Block J. Personality as an affect-processing system: toward an integrative theory. Mahwah (NJ): Lawrence Erlbaum; 2002.

[10] Achenbach TM, McConaughy SH. Empirically based assessment of child and adolescent psychopathology: practical applications. 2nd edition. Thousand Oaks (CA): Sage Publications, Inc.; 1997.

[11] Ivanova MY, Achenbach TM, Dumenci L, et al. Testing the 8-syndrome structure of the child behavior checklist in 30 societies. J Clin Child Adolesc Psychol 2007;36(3):405–17.

[12] Achenbach TM, Dumenci L, Rescorla LA. DSM-oriented and empirically based approaches to constructing scales from the same item pools. J Clin Child Adolesc Psychol 2003;32(3): 328–40.

[13] Coolidge FL, Thede LL, Jang KL. Heritability of personality disorders in childhood: a preliminary investigation. J Personal Disord 2001;15(1):33–40.

[14] Caspi A, Roberts BW, Shiner RL. Personality development: stability and change. Annu Rev Psychol 2005;56:453–84.

[15] Shiner RL. A developmental perspective on personality disorders: lessons from research on normal personality development in childhood and adolescence. J Personal Disord 2005;19(2):202–10.

[16] Rothbart MK, Ahadi SA, Hersey KL, et al. Investigations of temperament at three to seven years: the children's behavior questionnaire. Child Dev 2001;72(5):1394–408.

[17] Cohen P. Personality development in childhood: theoretical and empirical aspects. In: Cloninger HR, editor. Personality and psychopathology. Washington, DC: American Psychiatric Press; 1999. p. 101–27.

[18] Thomas A, Chess S. Temperament and development. New York: Brunner/Mazel; 1977.

[19] Digman JM. Higher-order factors of the big five. J Pers Soc Psychol 1997;73(6):1246–56.

[20] Bernstein DP, Cohen P, Skodol A, et al. Childhood antecedents of adolescent personality disorders. Am J Psychiatry 1996;153(7):907–13.

[21] Moffitt TE. Adolescence-limited and life-course-persistent antisocial behavior: a developmental taxonomy. Psychol Rev 1993;100(4):674–701.

[22] Loeber R, Burke JD, Lahey BB. What are adolescent antecedents to antisocial personality disorder? Crim Behav Ment Health 2002;12(1):24–36.

[23] Farrington DP. The importance of child and adolescent psychopathy. J Abnorm Child Psychol 2005;33(4):489–97.

[24] Loney BR, Frick PJ, Clements CB, et al. Callous-unemotional traits, impulsivity, and emotional processing in adolescents with antisocial behavior problems. J Clin Child Adolesc Psychol 2003;32(1):66–80.

[25] Jolliffe D, Farrington DP. Development and validation of the basic empathy scale. J Adolesc 2006;29(4):589–611.

[26] Salekin RT, Ziegler TA, Larrea MA, et al. Predicting dangerousness with two Millon Adolescent Clinical Inventory psychopathy scales: the importance of egocentric and callous traits. J Pers Assess 2003;80(2):154–63.

[27] Vasey MW, Kotov R, Frick PJ, et al. The latent structure of psychopathy in youth: a taxometric investigation. J Abnorm Child Psychol 2005;33(4):411–29.

[28] Salekin RT, Frick PJ. Psychopathy in children and adolescents: the need for a developmental perspective. J Abnorm Child Psychol 2005;33(4):403–9.

[29] Frick PJ, Kimonis ER, Dandreaux DM, et al. The 4 year stability of psychopathic traits in non-referred youth. Behav Sci Law 2003;21(6):713–36.

[30] Frick PJ, Stickle TR, Dandreaux DM, et al. Callous-unemotional traits in predicting the severity and stability of conduct problems and delinquency. J Abnorm Child Psychol 2005;33(4):471–87.

[31] Smith A. Cognitive empathy and emotional empathy in human behavior and evolution. Psychol Rec 2006;56(1):3–21.

[32] Symons DK. Mental state discourse, theory of mind, and the internalization of self-other understanding. Dev Rev 2004;24(2):159–88.

[33] Farrington DP. Building developmental and life-course theories of offending. In: Cullen FT, Wright JP, Blevins KR, editors. Taking stock: the status of criminological theory. New Brunswick (NJ): Transaction Publishers; 2006. p. 335–64.

[34] Crick NR, Murray-Close D, Woods K. Borderline personality features in childhood: a short-term longitudinal study. Dev Psychopathol 2005;17(4):1051–70.

[35] Rogosch FA, Cicchetti D. Child maltreatment, attention networks, and potential precursors to borderline personality disorder. Dev Psychopathol 2005;17(4):1071–89.

[36] Becker DF, Grilo CM, Edell WS, et al. Diagnostic efficiency of borderline personality disorder criteria in hospitalized adolescents: comparison with hospitalized adults. Am J Psychiatry 2002;159(12):2042–7.

[37] Becker DF, Grilo CM. Validation studies of the borderline personality disorder construct in adolescents. Adolesc Psychiatry 2006;29:217–35.

[38] Zelkowitz P, Paris J, Guzder J, et al. Diathesis and stressors in borderline pathology of childhood: the role of neuropsychological risk and trauma. J Am Acad Child Adolesc Psychiatry 2001;40(1):100–5.

[39] Westen D, Dutra L, Shedler J. Assessing adolescent personality pathology. Br J Psychiatry 2005;186(3):227–38.

[40] Westen D, Nakash O, Thomas C, et al. Clinical assessment of attachment patterns and personality disorder in adolescents and adults. J Consult Clin Psychol 2006;74(6):1065–85.

[41] Coolidge FL. Coolidge personality and neuropsychological inventory for children manual. Colorado Springs (CO): Author; 1998.

[42] Hyler SE, Oldham JM, Rosnick L. Validity of the Personality Diagnostic Questionnaire-Revised: Comparison with two structured interviews. American Journal of Psychiatry 1990;47:1043–8.

[43] Crawford TN, Cohen P, Johnson JG, et al. Self-reported personality disorder in the children in the community sample: convergent and prospective validity in late adolescence and adulthood. J Personal Disord 2005;19(1):30–52.

[44] Chen H, Cohen P, Crawford TN, et al. Relative impact of young adult personality disorders on subsequent quality of life: findings of a community-based longitudinal study. J Personal Disord 2006;20(5):510–23.

[45] De Clercq B, De Fruyt F. Childhood antecedents of personality disorder. Curr Opin Psychiatry 2007;20(1):57–61.

[46] Cohen P. Childhood risks for young adult symptoms of personality disorder: method and substance. Multivariate Behav Res 1996;31(1):121–48.

[47] Johnson JG, Cohen P, Brown J, et al. Childhood maltreatment increases risk for personality disorders during early adulthood. Arch Gen Psychiatry 1999;56(7):600–6.

[48] Cohen P, Chen H, Gordon K, et al. Socioeconomic background and the developmental course of schizotypal and borderline personality disorder symptoms. Dev Psychopathol 2008;20(2):633–50.

[49] Guzder J, Paris J, Zelkowitz P, et al. Psychological risk factors for borderline pathology in school-age children. J Am Acad Child Adolesc Psychiatry 1999;38(2):206–12.

[50] Neugebauer R, Hoek HW, Susser E. Prenatal exposure to wartime famine and development of antisocial personality disorder in early adulthood. J Am Med Assoc 1999;282(5):455–62.

[51] Waters HS, Waters E. The attachment working models concept: among other things, we build script-like representations of secure base experiences. Attach Hum Dev 2006;8(3):185–97.

[52] Bowlby J. Disruption of affectional bonds and its effects on behavior. J Contemporary Psychotherapy 1970;2(2):75–86.

[53] Crawford TN, Shaver PR, Cohen P, et al. Self-reported attachment, interpersonal aggression, and personality disorder in a prospective community sample of adolescents and adults. J Personal Disord 2006;20(4):331–51.

[54] Bezirganian S, Cohen P, Brook JS. The impact of mother-child interaction on the development of borderline personality disorder. Am J Psychiatry 1993;150(12):1836–42.

[55] Johnson JG, Cohen P, Chen H, et al. Parenting behaviors associated with risk for offspring personality disorder during adulthood. Arch Gen Psychiatry 2006;63(5):579–87.

[56] Johnson JG, Bromley E, McGeoch PG. Role of childhood experiences in the development of maladaptive and adaptive personality traits. In: Oldham JM, Skodol AE, Bender DS, editors. The American Psychiatric Publishing textbook of personality disorders. Washington, DC: American Psychiatric Publishing, Inc.; 2005. p. 209–21.

[57] Teicher MH, Tomoda A, Andersen SL. Neurobiological consequences of early stress and childhood maltreatment: are results from human and animal studies comparable? In: Yehuda R, editor. Psychobiology of posttraumatic stress disorders: a decade of progress, vol. 1071. Malden (MA): Blackwell Publishing; 2006. p. 313–23.

[58] Guzder J, Paris J, Zelkowitz P, et al. Risk factors for borderline pathology in children. J Am Acad Child Adolesc Psychiatry 1996;35(1):26–33.

[59] Paris J, Zelkowitz P, Guzder J, et al. Neuropsychological factors associated with borderline pathology in children. J Am Acad Child Adolesc Psychiatry 1999;38(6):770–4.

[60] Biederman J, Hirshfeld-Becker DR, Rosenbaum JF, et al. Further evidence of association between behavioral inhibition and social anxiety in children. Am J Psychiatry 2001;158(10):1673–9.

[61] Zanarini MC, Frankenburg FR, Ridolfi ME, et al. Reported childhood onset of self-mutilation among borderline patients. J Personal Disord 2006;20(1):9–15.

[62] Cohen P, Cohen J. Life values and adolescent mental health. Mahwah (NJ): Lawrence Erlbaum Assoc; 1997.

[63] Cohen P, Cohen J. Life values and mental health in adolescence. In: Schmuck P, Sheldon KM, editors. Life goals and well-being: towards a positive psychology of human striving. Ashland (OH): Hogrefe & Huber Publishers; 2001. p. 167–81.

[64] Mervielde I, De Clercq B, De Fruyt F, et al. Temperament, personality, and developmental psychopathology as childhood antecedents of personality disorders. J Personal Disord 2005;19(2):171–201.

[65] Van Leeuwen KG, Mervielde I, De Clerco BJ, et al. Extending the spectrum idea: child personality, parenting and psychopathology. European Journal of Personality 2007;21(1):63–89.

[66] Paris J. Personality disorders over time: precursors, course and outcome. J Personal Disord 2003;17(6):479–88.

[67] Helgeland MI, Kjelsberg E, Torgersen S. Continuities between emotional and disruptive behavior disorders in adolescence and personality disorders in adulthood. Am J Psychiatry 2005;162(10):1941–7.

[68] Bernstein DP, Cohen P, Velez CN, et al. Prevalence and stability of the DSM-III–R personality disorders in a community-based survey of adolescents. Am J Psychiatry 1993;150(8): 1237–43.

[69] Johnson JG, Cohen P, Kasen S, et al. Age-related change in personality disorder trait levels between early adolescence and adulthood: a community-based longitudinal investigation. Acta Psychiatr Scand 2000;102(4):265–75.

[70] Lenzenweger MF. Stability and change in personality disorder features: the longitudinal study of personality disorders. Arch Gen Psychiatry 1999;56(11):1009–15.

[71] Johnson JG, First MB, Cohen P, et al. Adverse outcomes associated with personality disorder not otherwise specified in a community sample. Am J Psychiatry 2005;162(10):1926–32.

[72] Hamagami F, McArdle JJ, Cohen P. A new approach to modeling bivariate dynamic relationships applied to evaluation of comorbidity among DSM-III personality disorder symptoms. In: Molfese VJ, Molfese DL, editors. Temperament and personality development across the life span. Mahwah (NJ): Lawrence Erlbaum Associates Publishers; 2000. p. 253–80.

[73] Becker DF, Grilo CM, Edell WS, et al. Comorbidity of borderline personality disorder with other personality disorders in hospitalized adolescents and adults. Am J Psychiatry 2000;157(12):2011–6.

[74] Crawford TN, Cohen P, First MB, et al. Comorbid axis I and axis II disorders in early adolescence: prognosis for 20 years later. Arch Gen Psychiatry 2008;65(6):in press.

[75] Kasen S, Cohen P, Skodol AE, et al. Influence of child and adolescent psychiatric disorders on young adult personality disorder. Am J Psychiatry 1999;156(10):1529–35.

[76] Kasen S, Cohen P, Skodol AE, et al. Childhood depression and adult personality disorder: alternative pathways of continuity. Arch Gen Psychiatry 2001;58(3):231–6.

[77] Goodwin RD, Brook JS, Cohen P. Panic attacks and the risk of personality disorder. Psychol Med 2005;35(2):227–35.

[78] Johnson JG, Cohen P, Kasen S, et al. Personality disorder traits associated with risk for unipolar depression during middle adulthood. Psychiatry Res 2005;136(2–3):113–21.

[79] Cohen P, Chen H, Crawford TN, et al. Personality disorders in early adolescence and the development of later substance use disorders in the general population. Drug Alcohol Depend 2007;88:S71–84.

[80] Kasen S, Cohen P, Skodol AE, et al. Comorbid personality disorder and treatment use in a community sample of youths: a 20-year follow-up. Acta Psychiatr Scand 2007;115(1): 56–65.

[81] Crawford TN, Cohen P, Johnson JG, et al. The course and psychosocial correlates of personality disorder symptoms in adolescence: Erikson's developmental theory revisited. J Youth Adolesc 2004;33(5):373–87.

[82] Johnson JG, Chen H, Cohen P. Personality disorder traits during adolescence and relationships with family members during the transition to adulthood. J Consult Clin Psychol 2004;72(6):923–32.

[83] Chen H, Cohen P, Kasen S, et al. Adolescent axis I and personality disorders predict quality of life during young adulthood. J Adolesc Health 2006;39(1):14–9.

[84] Cohen P, Chen H, Kasen S, et al. Adolescent cluster A personality disorder symptoms, role assumption in the transition to adulthood, and resolution or persistence of symptoms. Dev Psychopathol 2005;17(2):549–68.

[85] Ehrensaft MK, Cohen P, Johnson JG. Development of personality disorder symptoms and the risk for partner violence. J Abnorm Psychol 2006;115(3):474–83.

[86] Johnson JG, Cohen P, Smailes E, et al. Adolescent personality disorders associated with violence and criminal behavior during adolescence and early adulthood. Am J Psychiatry 2000;157:1406–12.

[87] Chen H, Cohen P, Johnson JG, et al. Adolescent personality disorders and conflict with romantic partners during the transition to adulthood. J Personal Disord 2004;18(6):507–25.

[88] Winograd G, Cohen P, Chen H. Adolescent borderline symptoms in the community: impact on functioning over 20 years. J Child Psychol Psychiatry 2008;48,in press.

Longitudinal Course and Outcome of Personality Disorders

Andrew E. Skodol, MD[a,b,*]

[a]Institute for Mental Health Research, 3300 N. Central Avenue, Suite 2380, Phoenix,
AZ 85012, USA
[b]University of Arizona College of Medicine, Phoenix, Arizona, USA

Personality disorders have been diagnosed (along with mental retardation) on a separate axis from other mental disorders ever since the creation of a multiaxial diagnostic format for the *Diagnostic and Statistical Manual of Mental Disorders, third edition* (DSM-III) in 1980. Originally, the rationale for disorders on Axis II was to ensure that they would be considered in the comprehensive diagnostic evaluation represented by the five-axis system. In DSM-III-R, the stated rationale for Axis II disorders changed: they were believed to "begin in childhood or adolescence and persist in stable form (without periods of remission or exacerbation) into adult life" [1]. The rationale for Axis II was changed again in DSM-IV to ensure that "consideration will given to the possible presence of Personality Disorders ... that might otherwise be overlooked when attention is directed to the usually more fluid Axis I disorders" [2], language reminiscent of the original wording in DSM-III.

Despite these shifts back and forth on the rationale for Axis II, the definition of personality disorder in DSM-IV (and DSM-IV-TR) continues to reflect the traditional view of personality disorders as enduring and stable over time. Criterion A of the general diagnostic criteria for a personality disorder in DSM-IV-TR refers to "an *enduring* pattern of inner experiences and behavior ... manifested in cognition, affectivity, interpersonal functioning, or impulse control." Criterion B states that "the *enduring* pattern is inflexible and pervasive." Criterion C requires that "the *enduring* pattern leads to clinically significant distress or impairment in ... functioning." Criteria D states that the "pattern is stable and of long duration." Criteria E and F indicate that "the *enduring* pattern is not better accounted for as a manifestation ... of another mental disorder" nor "due to ... a substance or a general medical condition" [3].

Thus, the notion of personality disorders as stable disorders to be distinguished from the more episodic mental disorders diagnosed on Axis I persisted despite a large number of traditional follow-up studies in the DSM-III and

*Institute for Mental Health Research, 3300 N. Central Avenue, Suite 2380, Phoenix, AZ 85012. *E-mail address*: askodol@imhr.org

0193-953X/08/$ – see front matter
doi:10.1016/j.psc.2008.03.010
© 2008 Elsevier Inc. All rights reserved.

DSM-III-R eras that showed that fewer than 50% of patients diagnosed with personality disorders retained these diagnoses over time [4–9]. These studies, however, had substantial methodological problems that preclude firm conclusions from being drawn from them including small sample sizes, unstandardized diagnostic assessments, inattention to establishing inter-rater reliability, lack of "blindness" to baseline diagnoses, reliance on only two assessment time points, typically short follow-up periods, insufficient characterization of co-occurring disorders and of treatment received, focus almost exclusively on either borderline or antisocial personality disorders, and lack of relevant comparison groups.

Because of the limitations of these studies and the constraints they placed on conclusions to be drawn about the natural history of personality disorder psychopathology, a new generation of rigorous follow-along studies in community, nonpatient, and patient populations was spawned. The purpose of these studies has been to examine the short- and long-term course and impact of personality psychopathology and to determine what about personality disorders is stable?

FOUR NATURALISTIC STUDIES OF CLINICAL COURSE

The results of four large-scale studies of the naturalistic course of personality disorders are reviewed in this article. The four studies are The Children in the Community Study (CICS) [10], The Longitudinal Study of Personality Disorders (LSPD) [11], The McLean Study of Adult Development (MSAD) [12], and The Collaborative Longitudinal Personality Disorders Study (CLPS) [13]. Course and outcome in these studies has been examined in six different ways: diagnoses; criteria, symptoms, or traits; psychosocial functioning; behavioral problems; quality of life; and course of co-occurring Axis I disorders. These studies were conducted on community (CICS), nonpatient (LSPD), and patient populations (MSAD and CLPS).

The Children in the Community Study

The CICS is a longitudinal study of a sample of approximately 800 children, who were originally recruited (with their mothers) in upstate New York in 1975, when they were between 1 and 10 years of age [10]. They have been followed now periodically for nearly 30 years. Originally, the study was designed to assess level of need for children's services in the community. When first followed-up in 1983, the focus of the study shifted to predictors of Axis I disorders in early adolescence, but an interest in the development of personality disorders in this age group also existed. Using various methods, personality disorders have been assessed four times: in 1983, when the children were at mean age 14; between 1985 and 1986, when they were at mean age 16; between 1991 and 1993, at mean age 22; and between 2001 and 2004, at mean age 33.

Course of personality disorder symptoms

Given the prevalence of personality disorders in the general population, too few adolescents met criteria for disorders to reliably obtain stability estimates.

Therefore, the CICS examined the stability of personality disorder traits and found that levels decreased by 48% between adolescence (age 14–16) and early adulthood (age 22) [14].

Impact on psychosocial functioning
The impact of personality disorder psychopathology on functioning has been examined in the CICS for each DSM personality disorder cluster. For cluster A (odd, eccentric cluster), adolescents with high symptom levels had lower education and achievement [15], greater partner conflict, and earlier childbearing [16] in early adulthood. Adolescents with high levels of cluster B (dramatic, erratic) symptoms had lower levels of intimacy [17] and sustained conflict with partners [16] in early adulthood. Adolescents with high levels of cluster C (anxious, fearful) symptoms had greater conflict with partners, if they had a partner [16]. Adolescents and young adults who qualified for a diagnosis of personality disorder not otherwise specified (PDNOS) experienced significant educational failure and interpersonal difficulties [18].

The effects of personality disorder stability on global functioning and impairment were also examined in the CICS [19]. Individuals with persistent personality disorders had markedly poorer functioning and greater impairment at mean age 33 than did those who had never been identified as having such a disorder or who had a personality disorder that was in remission. The effects of co-occurring Axis I disorders at age 33 were taken into account. Remitted personality disorders, ie, present before age 22, but not at age 33, was associated with mild long-term impairment. Adult-onset personality disorders (present at age 33, but not before) were also associated with significant impairment.

Impact on behavior
High levels of cluster A symptoms during adolescence predicted subsequent violent acts and criminal behavior [20]; high levels of cluster B symptoms predicted violent behavior [20]. In cluster C, adolescent dependent symptoms predicted suicidality [21]. Adolescents with PDNOS were also at risk for serious acts of aggression as young adults [18]. Young adult PD symptoms in all three clusters partially mediated violence against partners [22].

Impact on quality of life
Any personality disorder or any cluster A, B, or C personality disorder in early adulthood (age 22) was associated with reduced quality of life at age 33 [23]. Cluster B personality disorders had the greatest effect. Antisocial, borderline, and schizotypal symptoms were independently associated with quality of life reduction. These effects were independent of demographic characteristics, co-occurring Axis I disorders, and physical illnesses.

Impact on Axis I disorders
In cluster A personality disorders, adolescent or young adult symptoms increased risk of subsequent mood, eating, anxiety, and disruptive behavior disorders. Adolescent or young adult cluster B symptoms increased risk of subsequent mood, anxiety, eating, disruptive, *and* substance use disorders.

Cluster C symptoms increased risk of subsequent mood, anxiety, and disruptive behavior, but not eating or substance use, disorders [21,24–26].

The Longitudinal Study of Personality Disorders

The LSPD [11] is a multiwave, longitudinal study of Cornell University undergraduates. As such, it represents a study of personality psychopathology in individuals who were not identified patients, ie, not seeking treatment. Of 1684 eligible undergraduates, 258 were selected by screening and follow-up interviews. A total of 134 were identified as having probable personality disorders and 124 were deemed to have no personality disorder. These participants were then followed three times over a 4-year interval.

Course of personality disorder symptoms
Once again, because of the insufficient number of individual personality disorders at the categorical (threshold) level to allow analysis of the stability of disorders, personality disorder symptoms were examined as continuous dimensions. Personality disorder dimensions showed significant levels of stability, both by interview and self-report [27]. However, personality disorder features in this study also showed significant declines over time: personality psychopathology decreased by 1.4 features per year over 4 years [28]. Psychosocial functioning has not been measured in the LSPD to date, although its measurement is anticipated in future follow-along waves.

The McLean Study of Adult Development

The MSAD [12] is the first National Institute of Mental Health (NIMH)-funded prospective study of the course and outcome of borderline personality disorder (BPD). The MSAD sample consists of 290 patients with borderline personality disorder who were inpatients at McLean Hospital in the early 1990s and 72 other inpatients who were diagnosed with other personality disorders. This comparison group included approximately 4% with cluster A personality disorders, 18% with other nonborderline cluster B disorders, 33% with cluster C personality disorders, and 53% with PDNOS. The sample has been followed every 2 years for more than 12 years.

Course of personality disorder diagnoses
The most striking finding of the MSAD has been the degree of improvement in the patients with BPD: 88% of these patients experienced a remission within 10 years [29]. Furthermore, these remissions appear to be quite stable: only about 6% of the borderline patients had a recurrence.

Impact on psychosocial functioning
Overall, the psychosocial functioning of borderline patients in the MSAD improved significantly over the first 6 years of follow-up. Compared with only 26% of the borderline sample who were rated as having good or better functioning when recruited in the hospital, 56% were found to have at least good functioning 6 years later [30]. Nonetheless, borderline patients continued to function more poorly than patients with other personality disorders,

particularly in the area of vocational achievement. Borderline patients who experienced symptomatic remission functioned significantly better socially and vocationally than those who did not remit, eg, 66% with good functioning in the former group versus 27% in the latter group.

Impact on Axis I disorders
Patients with borderline personality disorder experienced declining rates of many Axis I disorders over 6 years [31]. Rates of mood and anxiety disorders continued to remain high, however. Consistent with the MSAD findings on effects of remission on functioning, patients with BPD who had a remission experienced declines in all comorbid disorders assessed, while those who did not remit reported stable rates.

Collaborative Longitudinal Personality Disorders Study

The CLPS [13] is a multisite, NIMH-funded longitudinal study of the natural course of personality disorders. Participating sites are at Brown, Columbia (now in collaboration with the Institute for Mental Health Research and the University of Arizona), Harvard, Yale, and Texas A & M universities. The aims of the CLPS have been to determine the stability of personality disorder diagnoses and criteria, personality traits, and functional impairment, and to determine the predictors of clinical course. The original CLPS sample recruited 668 treatment-seeking or recently treated patients who were diagnosed with one of four DSM-IV personality disorders—schizotypal, borderline, avoidant, or obsessive-compulsive—or with major depressive disorder and no personality disorder. This original sample was supplemented with the recruitment of 65 additional minority patients to ensure adequate power to test differences between Caucasian, African American, and Hispanic patients with the four personality disorders on various outcomes. The original CLPS sample is now in its 10th year of follow-up.

Course of personality disorder diagnoses and criteria
The CLPS study, like the MSAD, has found surprising rates of improvement in patients diagnosed with personality disorders. The CLPS has used two definitions of remission: meeting two or fewer criteria of a personality disorder diagnosis for 2 consecutive months and meeting two or fewer criteria for 12 consecutive months. The former definition was to allow for a direct comparison of personality disorder remission with the widely accepted definition used for major depressive disorder, the CLPS comparison group, and the latter definition was to provide for a more clinically significant indicator of improvement.

Within the first 2 years of follow-up, between 33% (schizotypal) and 55% (obsessive-compulsive) of patients with personality disorders experienced a period of remission according to the 2-month standard [32]. Between 23% (schizotypal) and 38% (obsessive-compulsive) experienced a 12-month remission. In addition, on blind retest at 2 years, between 50% and 60% were below the threshold for a personality disorder diagnosis. The mean proportion of criteria met declined significantly for each of the personality disorders. These patterns of criteria decline and rates of remission have continued over the first 6 years of follow-up, such that by year 6, over three fourths of patients with personality disorders have had a 2-month remission and over two thirds have had a 12-month remission (Skodol, unpublished data, 2008). Relapses have also occurred, however, within the first 6 years. Relapse rates vary by personality disorder diagnosis: schizotypal personality disorder has had the lowest relapse rates and avoidant personality disorder has had the highest relapse rates.

When viewed as continuous dimensions, counts of the number of criteria met correlated with baseline counts 0.74 at 6 months, 0.67 at 1 year, and 0.59 at 2 years [32]. These correlations are very similar to correlations of personality traits across age categories represented in the CLPS (18 to 45 years) as reported in a meta-analysis of 152 longitudinal studies by Roberts and Del Vecchio [33].

Predictors of change in personality disorders include changes in traits of general personality functioning [34], as well as changes in certain Axis I disorders (eg, major depressive disorder and posttraumatic stress disorder for borderline personality disorder and social phobia for avoidant personality disorder) [35]. The Axis I/Axis II change effects were shown to be reciprocal and not unidirectional, however.

Impact on behavior
During the first 2 years of follow-up, 9% of study participants reported at least one definitive suicide attempt and 44% of these had multiple suicidal behaviors [36]. Suicide attempts were more common in borderline patients and in those with drug use disorders. Twelve percent of personality disordered patients attempted suicide by the 3-year follow-up [37].

Impact of psychosocial functioning
Despite the significant remission rates and declines in criteria counts found in the CLPS, functional impairment has remained remarkably stable. For example, ratings on the Global Assessment of Functioning Scale (Axis V: GAFS) did not change significantly for any of the four personality disorders in the first 2 years of follow-up; only functioning in the major depressive disorder group improved [38]. These results have also held up at the 4-year follow-up (Skodol, unpublished data, 2008). In a comparison of the ability of diagnostic models, including DSM-IV dimensions, the Five-Factor Model, and a Three-Factor Model, to predict functioning (and other external validators) over time, the DSM-IV relationships were strongest at the baseline assessment and declined over 4 years, while the trait-based models were less predictive at baseline, but more predictive over time [39,40]. This suggests that the DSM-IV representation of personality psychopathology does capture important variance in functioning when patients have acute problems and are seeking treatment, but that over the natural course of personality disorder, traits capture variance in functioning better than DSM-IV. A hybrid model consisting of more stable, temperamental traits and less stable, situationally dependent symptomatic behaviors

may be the best representation of personality disorder and should be considered for DSM-V [41].

Impact on Axis I disorders

The time to remission of episodes of major depressive disorder in the CLPS sample has been shown to be longer when a patient also has a personality disorder [42]. By 2 years, 90% of depressed patients without a personality disorder have remitted, compared with approximately two thirds with at least one personality disorder. The presence or severity of personality disorder was not found to affect the course of eating disorders, however [43].

SUMMARY

The results of these four rigorous studies of the naturalistic course of personality disorders indicate the following: (1) personality psychopathology improves over time at unexpectedly significant rates; (2) maladaptive personality traits are more stable than personality disorder diagnoses; (3) although personality psychopathology improves, residual effects are usually seen in the form of persistent functional impairment, continuing behavioral problems, reduced future quality of life, and ongoing Axis I psychopathology; and (4) improvement in personality psychopathology may eventually be associated with reduction in ongoing personal and social burden.

Personality psychopathology may be more waxing and waning than traditionally thought. Because personality disorders have their origins in childhood or adolescence, deficits in the development of affect regulation, conscience, impulse control, or identity consolidation can be expected to have adverse and persistent effects on a person's adaptation to the occupational and social demands of young adult life. More attention should be paid in treatment and research to the long-term negative consequences of personality disorders.

References

[1] American Psychiatric Association. Diagnostic and statistical manual of mental disorders. Revised (DSM-III-R). 3rd edition. Washington, DC: American Psychiatric Association; 1987. p. 16.
[2] American Psychiatric Association. Diagnostic and statistical manual of mental disorders. (DSM-IV). 4th edition. Washington, DC: American Psychiatric Association; 1994. p. 26.
[3] American Psychiatric Association. Diagnostic and statistical manual of mental disorders text revision. 4th edition. Washington, DC: American Psychiatric Association; 2000. p. 689.
[4] Perry JC. Longitudinal studies of personality disorders. J Personal Disord 1993;7(Suppl): 63–85.
[5] Zimmerman M. Diagnosing personality disorders: a review of issues and research methods. Arch Gen Psychiatry 1994;51(3):225–45.
[6] McDavid JD, Pilkonis PA. The stability of personality disorder diagnoses. J Personal Disord 1996;10(1):1–15.
[7] Grilo CM, McGlashan TH, Oldham JM. Course and stability of personality disorders. J Pract Psychiatry Behav Health 1998;4:61–75.
[8] Grilo CM, McGlashan TH. Stability and course of personality disorders. Curr Opin Psychiatry 1999;12:157–62.
[9] Paris J. Personality disorders over time: precursors, course and outcome. J Personal Disord 2003;17(6):479–88.

[10] Cohen P, Crawford TN, Johnson JG, et al. The children in the community study of developmental course of personality disorder. J Personal Disord 2005;19(5):466–86.

[11] Lenzenweger MF. The longitudinal study of personality disorders: history, design considerations, and initial findings. J Personal Disord 2006;20(6):645–70.

[12] Zanarini MC, Frankenburg FR, Hennen J, et al. The McLean study of adult development (MSAD): overview and implications of the first six years of prospective follow-up. J Personal Disord 2005;19(5):505–23.

[13] Skodol AE, Gunderson JG, Shea MT, et al. The collaborative longitudinal personality disorders study (CLPS): overview and implications. J Personal Disord 2005;19(5):487–504.

[14] Johnson JG, Cohen P, Kasen S, et al. Age-related change in personality disorder trait levels between early adolescence and adulthood: a community-based longitudinal investigation. Acta Psychiatr Scand 2000;102(4):265–75.

[15] Cohen P, Chen H, Kasen S, et al. Adolescent cluster A personality disorder symptoms, role assumption in the transition to adulthood, and resolution or persistence of symptoms. Dev Psychopathol 2005;17(2):549–68.

[16] Chen H, Cohen P, Johnson JG, et al. Adolescent personality disorder and conflict with romantic partners during the transition to adulthood. J Personal Disord 2004;18(6):507–25.

[17] Crawford TN, Cohen P, Johnson JG, et al. The course and psychosocial correlates of personality disorder symptoms in adolescence: Erickson's developmental theory revisited. J Youth Adolesc 2004;33:373–87.

[18] Johnson JG, First MB, Cohen P, et al. Adverse outcomes associated with personality disorder not otherwise specified (PDNOS) in a community sample. Am J Psychiatry 2005;162(10):1926–32.

[19] Skodol AE, Johnson JG, Cohen P, et al. Personality disorder and impaired functioning from adolescence to adulthood. Br J Psychiatry 2007;190:415–20.

[20] Johnson JG, Cohen P, Smailes E, et al. Adolescent personality disorders associated with violence and criminal behavior during adolescence and early adulthood. Am J Psychiatry 2000;157(9):1406–12.

[21] Johnson JG, Cohen P, Skodol AE, et al. Personality disorders in adolescence and risk of major mental disorders and suicidality during adulthood. Arch Gen Psychiatry 1999;56(9):805–11.

[22] Ehrensaft MK, Cohen P, Johnson JG. Development of personality disorder symptoms and the risk for partner violence. J Abnorm Psychol 2006;115(3):474–83.

[23] Chen H, Cohen P, Crawford TN, et al. Relative impact of young adult personality disorders on subsequent quality of life: findings of a community-based longitudinal study. J Personal Disord 2006;20(5):510–23.

[24] Johnson JG, Cohen P, Kasen S, et al. Personality disorder traits associated with risk for unipolar depression during middle adulthood. Psychiatry Res 2005;136(2–3):113–21.

[25] Johnson JG, Cohen P, Kasen S, et al. Personality disorders evident by early adulthood and risk for eating and weight problems during middle adulthood. Int J Eat Disord 2006;39(3):184–92.

[26] Johnson JG, Cohen P, Kasen S, et al. Personality disorder traits evident by early adulthood and risk for anxiety disorders during middle adulthood. J Anxiety Disord 2006;20(4):408–26.

[27] Lenzenweger MF. Stability and change in personality disorder features. Arch Gen Psychiatry 1999;56(11):1009–15.

[28] Lenzenweger MR, Johnson MD, Willett JB. Individual growth curve analysis illuminates stability and change in personality disorder features: The Longitudinal Study of Personality disorders. Arch Gen Psychiatry 2004;61(10):1015–24.

[29] Zanarini MC, Frankenburg FR, Hennen J, et al. Prediction of the 10-year course of borderline personality disorder. Am J Psychiatry 2006;163(5):827–32.

[30] Zanarini MC, Frankenburg FR, Hennen J, et al. Psychosocial functioning of borderline patients and Axis II comparison subjects followed prospectively for six years. J Personal Disord 2005;19(1):19–29.

[31] Zanarini MC, Frankenburg FR, Hennen J, et al. Axis I comorbidity of borderline personality disorder: description of six-year course and prediction of time-to-remission. Am J Psychiatry 2004;161(11):2108–14.

[32] Grilo CM, Shea MT, Sanislow CA, et al. Two-year stability and change in schizotypal, borderline, avoidant and obsessive-compulsive personality disorders. J Consult Clin Psychol 2004;72(5):767–75.

[33] Roberts BW, Del Vecchio WF. The rank-order consistency of personality traits from childhood to old age: a quantitative review of longitudinal studies. Psychol Bull 2000;126(1): 3–25.

[34] Warner MB, Morey LC, Finch JF, et al. The longitudinal relationship of personality traits and disorders. J Abnorm Psychol 2004;113(2):217–27.

[35] Shea MT, Stout RL, Yen S, et al. Associations in the course of personality disorders and Axis I disorders over time. J Abnorm Psychol 2004;113(4):499–508.

[36] Yen S, Shea MT, Pagano M, et al. Axis I and Axis II disorders as predictors of prospective suicide attempts: findings from the Collaborative Longitudinal Personality Disorders Study. J Abnorm Psychol 2003;112(3):375–81.

[37] Yen S, Pagano ME, Shea MT, et al. Recent life events preceding suicide attempts in a personality disorder sample: findings from the Collaborative Longitudinal Personality Disorders Study. J Consult Clin Psychol 2005;73(1):99–105.

[38] Skodol AE, Pagano ME, Bender DS, et al. Stability of functional impairment in patients with schizotypal, borderline, avoidant, or obsessive-compulsive personality disorder over two years. Psychol Med 2005;35(3):443–51.

[39] Skodol AE, Oldham JM, Bender DS, et al. Dimensional representations of DSM-IV personality disorders: relationships to functional impairment. Am J Psychiatry 2005;162(10): 1919–25.

[40] Morey LC, Hopwood CJ, Gunderson JG, et al. Comparison of alternative models for personality disorders. Psychol Med 2007;37:983–94.

[41] McGlashan TH, Grilo CM, Sanislow CA, et al. Two-year prevalence and stability of individual criteria for schizotypal, borderline, avoidant, and obsessive-compulsive personality disorders: toward a hybrid model of Axis II disorders. Am J Psychiatry 2005;162(5):883–9.

[42] Grilo CM, Sanislow CA, Shea MT, et al. Two-year prospective naturalistic study of remission from major depressive disorder as a function of personality disorder co-morbidity. J Consult Clin Psychol 2005;73(1):78–85.

[43] Grilo CM, Sanislow CA, Shea MT, et al. The natural course of bulimia nervosa and eating disorder not otherwise specified is not influenced by personality disorders. Int J Eat Disord 2003;34(3):319–30.

Psychiatr Clin N Am 31 (2008) 505–515

PSYCHIATRIC CLINICS
OF NORTH AMERICA

ELSEVIER
SAUNDERS

Reasons for Change in Borderline Personality Disorder (and Other Axis II Disorders)

Mary C. Zanarini, EdD

Laboratory for the Study of Adult Development, McLean Hospital and Harvard Medical School, 115 Mill Street, Belmont, MA 02478, USA

B orderline personality disorder (BPD) was long thought to be a chronic condition that affected most—or at least many—parts of a person's personality and functioning. Recent research has found that change is to be expected for many patients who have BPD over time—both in the symptomatic and psychosocial realms. More specifically, two large-scale studies prospectively studied the longitudinal course of BPD [1,2]. The longer running of these studies—the McLean Study of Adult Development (MSAD)—has published findings pertaining to the 10-year course of BPD [3,4]. The shorter running of these studies—the Collaborative Longitudinal Personality Disorders Study (CLPS)—has published findings pertaining to the 4-year course of BPD [5,6].

SYMPTOMATIC CHANGE

In terms of symptomatic outcome, the MSAD study found that remissions are common and recurrences are relatively rare. More specifically, 88% of the subjects in the MSAD study experienced a remission of their BPD by the time of their 10-year follow-up, but less than 20% experienced a recurrence of BPD [3]. Equally importantly, the MSAD study found that half of the 24 symptoms of BPD studied could be called acute symptoms and half could be called temperamental symptoms [4]. In this view, acute symptoms remit relatively rapidly, are the best markers for the disorder, and are often the main reason for costly forms of psychiatric treatment, such as inpatient stays and day programs. For these reasons, it has been suggested that acute symptoms are akin to the positive symptoms of schizophrenia. In contrast, temperamental symptoms remit relatively slowly, are not specific to BPD, and are associated with ongoing psychosocial impairment. For these reasons, it has been suggested that temperamental symptoms are akin to the negative symptoms of schizophrenia.

Supported by NIMH grants MH47588 and MH62169.

E-mail address: zanarini@mclean.harvard.edu

Some acute symptoms reflect areas of core impulsivity, such as self-mutilation and suicide attempts. Other acute symptoms, such as stormy relationships or problems with devaluation/manipulation/sadism, involve active attempts to manage interpersonal difficulties. Temperamental symptoms also tend to fall into two groups. The first group involves chronic feelings of dysphoria, such as anger or loneliness/emptiness. The second group involves interpersonal symptoms that reflect abandonment or dependency issues, such as intolerance of aloneness or counterdependency problems.

It is important to note that 10-year MSAD findings concerning the symptomatic course of BPD have been confirmed by the 2-year results of the CLPS study. The MSAD finding that symptomatic improvement is common was confirmed [7,8], as was our finding of two types of borderline symptoms [9]. In the CLPS study, acute symptoms are called symptomatic behaviors and temperamental symptoms are called traits.

PSYCHOSOCIAL CHANGE

The MSAD study found that the psychosocial functioning of many patients who have BPD improved with time, with more of them reporting a life partner, children, friends, good relationship with a parent, and the ability to work and/or attend school effectively and in a sustained manner as the years progressed [10]. Their social functioning was better than their vocational functioning, however. Axis II comparison subjects also showed a higher level of vocation adaptation than patients who have BPD. In contrast, the results of the CLPS study suggested that the psychosocial functioning of many patients who have BPD does not improve much with time, particularly in the social realm [11]. The results of this study also suggested that the psychosocial functioning of borderline patients is less adaptive than that of depressed comparison subjects (who have no substantial axis II psychopathology).

PSYCHIATRIC TREATMENT

The results of the MSAD study suggested that treatment over time is the rule rather than the exception for patients who have BPD [12]. Even after 10 years of follow-up, approximately 70% of patients who have BPD (and 45% of axis II comparison subjects) reported being in individual psychotherapy and taking standing medications. They also reported high rates of aggressive polypharmacy, with 40% taking three or more standing medications, 20% taking four or more, and 10% taking five or more. Not surprisingly, this high rate of polypharmacy has been linked in this sample to a high rate of obesity and obesity-related illnesses [13].

In contrast, patients who had BPD in the CLPS study reported using declining rates of outpatient treatment, with 64% reporting being in therapy and 68% reporting taking medications after 3 years of follow-up [14]. Comparable MSAD figures at 2-year follow-up were 94% and 86%, respectively.

CORE PROBLEM OF BORDERLINE PERSONALITY DISORDER

Several models of borderline psychopathology have been suggested by leading theorists in the field. Linehan [15] suggested that BPD is best understood as a disorder of emotional dysregulation. In this model, the quick reactivity of patients who have BPD (and the lack of strategies to handle this deficit) is the core feature of BPD. Gunderson [16] suggested that BPD is best understood as a disorder of attachment. In this model, fears of abandonment and being alone are the core conflicts from which patients who have BPD suffer and are the most salient features of the disorder.

We believe that there are two key features of BPD, the first of which is the intense inner pain with which patients live on a chronic basis. This pain is distinguished from the pain of others by its multifaceted nature and overall amplitude [17]. It consists of dysphoric affects (eg, I feel grief stricken, I feel completely panicked) and dysphoric (or distorted) cognitions (eg, like I'm being tortured, like I am damaged beyond repair) that are specific to BPD. More recently, another group [18] also found that severe inner pain is characteristic and distinguishing for patients who have BPD.

The second feature, which is perhaps better known to clinicians, is the awkward nature of the efforts that patients who have BPD make to hide this pain and express it. Some of these efforts are behavioral or impulsive in nature. The most troubling impulse action patterns are self-mutilation and help-seeking suicide threats and gestures. Substance abuse, promiscuity, and disordered eating are also common and ultimately destructive in nature. Other efforts to obtain needed comfort and support are interpersonal, including such maladaptive patterns as devaluation, manipulation, and being demanding. Although the impulsive acts tend to frighten clinicians, these interpersonal patterns tend to anger them. Inexperienced clinicians often think of them as forms of misbehavior. We think it is less pejorative and more accurate to describe them as outmoded survival strategies.

Two key questions emerge. First, what causes the intense inner pain of patients who have BPD? Second, why do they handle it in such a self-defeating manner? In terms of the first question, we assumed approximately a decade ago that only serious adversity, such as childhood abuse and neglect, would result in the intense inner pain that characterizes and distinguishes patients who have BPD from patients in other diagnostic groups [19]. We currently believe that many patients who have BPD are so temperamentally vulnerable that much more subtle experiences can engender the suffering that they insist that others pay attention to and of which they are so ashamed.

Attempting to be more specific, we have suggested that their temperament could be conceptualized as being hyperbolic in nature [19]. In this view, patients who have BPD are uncommonly insistent and persistent that the intensity of their inner pain be recognized and acknowledged by others on whom they depend, such as family members, spouses, and mental health care professionals. Statements such as, "I am in the worse pain since the history of the world began" are not uncommon and suggest how isolated and alienated many patients who have BPD feel.

The question arises as to why patients who have BPD rely on interpersonal strategies that are so counterproductive? Why do they have such difficulty being straightforward and simply asking directly for support and comfort they so desperately seek and genuinely seem to need? There is no clear answer for these questions and not one backed up by much data. It seems likely, however, that much of the problem has arisen from the long latency between this tremendous burden of inner pain first arising in late latency or early adolescence and the cognitive map of a borderline diagnosis not being applied until a decade or more latter [20]. Child psychiatrists and psychologists often mistakenly believe that the DSM-IV system prevents them from giving someone under the age of 18 a diagnosis of BPD. Even more perplexing is the tendency of many mental health professionals to resist giving an adult patient, albeit often a young adult, a diagnosis of BPD because of the mistaken belief that it is a hopelessly chronic condition. In these cases, often diagnosis is not mentioned or a co-occurring condition becomes the focus of treatment. Sometimes the co-occurring disorder is one from which the patient actually suffers. Other times, however, the patient is aggressively treated for a disorder, such as bipolar disorder, which the patient never manifested.

In the ideal world, parents and their preborderline child would be told of the borderline diagnosis and learn all of the latest information about the condition, including the fact that it has a relatively good prognosis. This would short-circuit the process of harmfully self-destructive behavioral or interpersonal strategies from developing or at least interrupt their hardening into reflexive reactions to less than optimal parental responses to their child's pain and distress.

Put more simply, most children who develop full-blown cases of BDP do try to tell their parents of their anguish and misery. Often their parents downplay the seriousness of their complaints. Rather then realizing their parents are doing their best, many patients who have BPD believe that their parents do not love them because they are less-than-perfect children or their parents derive pleasure from their suffering. In our experience, parents often fail to recognize their child's suffering and fragility because of their own limitations, but rarely are they deliberately malevolent.

Compounding this scenario is the fact that patients who have BPD are often perceptive but lack insight. They tend to believe that they are masterful in conveying their distress, which unfortunately is not true. They also tend to be oblivious to the covert reproaches that they make of the behavior of others— that they are mean or selfish or totally self-absorbed. They see themselves as truth tellers when in reality they are behaving in a self-righteous manner that can offend and enrage others.

PSYCHOSOCIAL TREATMENTS

Currently, there are four comprehensive psychotherapies with some proven efficacy for the treatment of BPD or at least some of its symptoms. Two of these treatments are cognitive behavioral in nature: dialectical behavioral therapy [21] and schema-focused therapy [22]. The other two treatments are psychodynamic in nature: mentalization-based therapy [23] and transference-focused psychotherapy [24]. All of these treatments require at least a year of treatment and highly trained clinicians.

Dialectical behavioral therapy is the only one of these treatments to have its findings replicated multiple times [25]. It is also the only one to have numerous adherents in the United States. It is costly to provide, however, because it involves skills groups, individual therapy, and a consultation team that consists of at least several providers. For this reason, most sites that provide a dialectical behavioral therapy program provide a less intensive version of dialectical behavioral therapy than that suggested by Linehan— dialectical behavioral therapy–like treatment. The reality is that most patients who have BPD do not receive a manualized form of psychotherapy that has proven efficacy. Rather, they receive treatment that is eclectic in nature. It is our experience that this type of treatment, which in itself is difficult to find and pay for, is probably "good enough" for most patients who have BPD who are neither desperately ill inpatients nor chronic outpatients.

PHARMACOLOGICAL TREATMENTS

The results of 21 randomized double-blind, placebo, or comparator-controlled trials have been published or presented [26]. Six studies have assessed the efficacy of antidepressants (phenelzine [$n = 1$], tranylcypromine [$n = 1$], amitriptyline [$n = 1$], fluoxetine [$n = 2$], and fluvoxamine [$n = 1$]). Nine have assessed the efficacy of mood stabilizers (carbamazepine [$n = 1$], valproate [$n = 3$], topiramate [$n = 3$], lamotrigine [$n = 1$], and omega-3 fatty acids [$n = 1$]). Eleven have assessed the efficacy of antipsychotics (trifluoperazine [$n = 1$], haloperidol [$n = 2$], aripiprazole [$n = 1$], risperidone [$n = 1$], and olanzapine [$n = 6$]). In general, each of these classes of medication has been found to be somewhat efficacious. They also have been found to affect overlapping symptom domains. Not surprisingly, however, none has been found to be curative. Rather, all but one (risperidone) seem to take the edge off BPD. This is no small achievement but is not the magic bullet for which some clinicians hope.

PATHWAYS TO FEELING BETTER AND FUNCTIONING MORE EFFECTIVELY

Three things need to happen for the symptoms of a patient who has BPD to lessen in intensity and for a patient who have BPD to begin to function more effectively in the psychosocial realm. The first is to help the patient find a way to lessen his or her subjective inner pain, which can be of tremendous intensity and highly disabling. The second is to help the patient find a way to be more straightforward and direct in expressing his or her wishes or needs. The third is to help the patient find a way to be more future oriented and less obsessed with the past and its many disappointments.

LESSENING THE PAIN OF PATIENTS WHO HAVE BORDERLINE PERSONALITY DISORDER

What Linehan termed "validation" is an essential aspect of efforts to help lessen the pain of BPD. Patients need to feel that someone understands their pain and is neither frightened nor disgusted by it. This type of acceptance can come from a therapist, a friend, or a romantic partner. This ability to listen and empathize can be distorted in nonuseful or even destructive ways, however. In the process of acceptance of what can seem like unending pain, some companions can begin to convey an acceptance of the patients' "theory of the case" or the maladaptive ways in which the patients have handled their pain. This is less than fortunate because it interferes with patients' ability to forgive themselves and those who have disappointed or frustrated them. This type of inappropriate acceptance is also less than fortunate because it may serve to "harden" maladaptive behaviors, such as being excessively dependent on others or extortionate with them.

Although validation can halt the slide into ever deeper and perhaps dangerous levels of painful feelings and cognitions, it does not by itself lessen the pain of having BPD. Some of this pain is the result of failed attempts to live as a competent adult in the real world, where failure and lack of support are real options for everyone. Much of the pain that patients who have BPD experience is caused by less-than-perfect parenting of a temperamentally vulnerable child and adolescent. This might be thought of as primary pain; however, a good portion of this pain is secondary in nature and the result of unsuccessful efforts to make friends, find a life partner, or establish a record as a competent adult in the vocational realm.

For most patients who are still functioning in the world of work or school, every effort should be made to support their continuing in these adult roles. For patients who have recently given up this level of functioning, every effort should be made to support their often wavering and ambivalent determination to return to work or school, even on a part-time basis. Perhaps the worst thing that a mental health care professional or family member can do is to encourage or even insist that a patient go on social security disability. Although this is often ostensibly done to get the patient the accompanying federal health insurance that comes with being disabled, it often signals to the patient that people are giving up on him or her and expect only the adaptation of a chronic patient. Once this role is accepted, it becomes a herculean task to help the patient move toward a more autonomous stance. This task is not impossible, however, and needs to become a condition for the therapy to continue.

Much the same process can and should occur in the social realm, where there are three different types of relationships to maintain or attain: friendships with peers, relationships with parents and siblings, and relationships with romantic partners. Many patients who have BPD have a history of relatively good relationships with peers. Relationships with parents and romantic partners are often much more problematic, however. Many patients have conflictual relationships with their parents, others have relationships marked by neglect and distance, and some have relationships that oscillate between being chaotic and disengaged. Many patients who have BPD who have romantic partners have stormy relationships with them, oscillating between being needy and fleeing from the pain of honest intimacy.

Many patients who have BPD blame their parents for their difficulties. They also may blame their romantic partners and spouses, which is often far easier than accepting responsibility for one's own failures. Many patients who have BPD have such a negative self-view and such a harsh superego that they cannot see that failure is about having difficulty completing a task and not an indictment of one's entire being. One can have trouble functioning without being a bad person who should be dead.

LEARNING TO BE MORE STRAIGHTFORWARD

In our experience, clarifications are the best therapeutic technique to comfort patients who have BPD (or validate their pain). Clarifications are also the best therapeutic technique to help patients who have BPD learn to be more straightforward and direct in expressing their wishes or needs. Rather than aggressively confronting a patient about being devaluative, one might say, "Sometimes it is hard to believe that anyone is actually willing and able to help." This type of statement reflects the desperation that the patient was trying to convey without confronting his or her shaky self-esteem. It also conveys that language can be useful and direct, which is important because BPD is, in part, a language disorder. Clinicians who can translate quickly what seems like (or is) a reproach into a statement of distress that the patient thought he or she was making are able to maintain the emotional tone of the relationship. This type of intervention needs to be repeated often before a patient who has BPD begins to "get it."

Vocational responsibilities and relationships also can be helpful in teaching a patient who has BPD to be more straightforward. Work and school often can be laboratories in which a patient who has BPD who is not acutely overwhelmed with negative feelings can observe which interpersonal strategies are rewarded and which lead to undesired negative consequences, such as being criticized or fired. It is also an arena that makes it plain that life is unfair—something most patients who have BPD know in theory but do not believe applies to them.

Relationships also can be helpful in comforting patients who have BPD and helping them to learn to be more direct in dealing with other people. This is particularly so if the family member, friend, or romantic partner is somewhat more mature than the patient in question. Such a person may have compassion for a person who has BPD and realize that he or she is doing his or her best at that moment in time. Such a person also may be helpful in setting an example of how to be more direct. If a patient has been critical but does not seem to realize it, such a friend might say, "I don't think you know it but you are hurting my feelings. I wish you would stop so that we can be as close as we usually are." Such a comment captures the attention of someone who has BPD without seeming like an unfair or unbearable criticism. Chances are that the statement will be perceived as a useful piece of information that is meant to be helpful. Such comments are clarifications. In our experience, patients who have BPD first learn from friends. Then they make peace with their family members. Only with this level of support are they able to establish an enduring relationship with a romantic partner.

Patients who have BPD and have been sexually abused often believe that they can never have an intimate relationship, and some therapists support this position. There is no doubt that such a history can make a sexual adjustment difficult—with some patients avoiding sexual intimacy, others becoming symptomatic after having sex, and yet others suffering from both reactions [27]. It is difficult to deny, however, that the emotional intimacy of a relationship with a reasonable and committed life partner can help to assuage the wounds of BPD. In many ways, the comfort and instruction that a patient who has BPD wants and needs are better provided by individuals without a professional relationship to the patient. They have chosen to be close and are not being paid to spend time with the patient. They can and do expect a reciprocal relationship with the patient—one in which power is often not a particularly pressing issue.

Experience suggests that therapy is best thought of as being adjunctive to life and not a substitute for it. This thinking goes against what many mental health care professionals believe. In this view, therapy is essential to lay the groundwork for a better, less painful life. In some cases, therapy even turns into a lifestyle and is the most important element in a patient's life. We share the belief that therapy can and often does encourage and facilitate change. We also share the belief that it can be essential in helping to consolidate changes in the patient's life. We believe more strongly than many observers, however, that adult life offers patients who have BPD reparations for the hurt and adversities that they have endured.

TOWARD A FUTURE ORIENTATION

There is no denying that many patients who have BPD are attached to their past and have a difficult time seeing the value of or even the possibility of a forward-leaning orientation. This is so for two reasons. First (and less important) is the fact that many patients who have BPD are bitter about the pain they have had to endure and angry at the people (often their parents) who they believe did not do enough to alleviate their suffering. In time and with the help of their friends (and treaters), they may come to the realization that each of us only gets one childhood and no one can change the past. With an acceptance of life as it has played out for them and the realization that their parents did what they could come grief and the energy to pursue a real life in the real world.

The second (and more important) reason for their devotion to the past is that their pain represents—to a large extent—lost loves that have gone awry. It is part of their identity and they are afraid that it will never end and that it will end too soon. Looked at another way, most patients who have BPD were not unloved but loved in a manner that was too inconsistent for them. They are reluctant to give up the search for the "restoration" that they believe will make them whole. They look for this restoration in all the wrong places, including assuming that their therapist is withholding emotional supplies from them that are definitely curative in nature.

The best strategy for dealing with their initial lack of interest in a future is to encourage them to "get a life." Plainly, real life can offer better reparations than the limited but important relationship that patients can have with their therapist. These reparations bring with them the real possibility of new heartache, however. They also offer the real possibility of a "restoration" of some kind of peace and comfort that can only come with accepting life on its own terms. In the end, there is no point to "bargaining" with life because the "rules" of life apply equally to all of us. Trying to "wring" reparations from unwilling and unwitting others because of prior adversity is only a path to defeat and humiliation.

OTHER PERSONALITY DISORDERS

Antisocial personality disorder is the only other personality disorder that has been validated according to the rigorous criteria of Robins and Guze [28]. Patients who have antisocial personality disorder have been found to make progress over time [29]. It is not clear how these processes of change occur, however. The CLPS study also found that patients who have schizotypal, avoidant, and obsessive-compulsive personality disorders make symptomatic progress [7,8]. Again, it is not clear why this progress occurs.

SUMMARY

Most people who meet criteria for BPD change slowly over time. Although researchers have developed comprehensive psychosocial treatments for BPD, most patients improve with the help of treatment as usual and the support and guidance of persons who care about them. The evidence suggests that BPD is a good prognosis diagnosis. Although these individuals can be difficult and challenging, they deserve our respect for their struggles to achieve a better and less painful adaptation to the life they were given.

References

[1] Zanarini MC, Frankenburg FR, Hennen J, et al. The McLean Study of Adult Development (MSAD): overview and implications of the first six years of prospective follow-up. J Personal Disord 2005;19:505–23.

[2] Skodol AE, Gunderson JG, Shea MT, et al. The collaborative longitudinal personality disorders study: overview and implications. J Personal Disord 2005;19:487–504.

[3] Zanarini MC, Frankenburg FR, Hennen J, et al. Prediction of the 10-year course of borderline personality disorder. Am J Psychiatry 2006;163:827–32.

[4] Zanarini MC, Frankenburg FR, Reich DB, et al. The subsyndromal phenomenology of borderline personality disorder: a 10-year follow-up study. Am J Psychiatry 2007;164: 929–35.

[5] Gunderson JG, Weinberg I, Daversa MT, et al. Description and longitudinal observations on the relationship between borderline personality disorder and bipolar disorder. Am J Psychiatry 2006;163:1173–8.

[6] Skodol AE, Bender DS, Pagano ME, et al. Positive childhood experiences: resilience and recovery from personality disorder in early adulthood. J Clin Psychiatry 2007;68:1102–8.

[7] Shea MT, Stout RL, Gunderson JG, et al. Short-term diagnostic stability of schizotypal, borderline, avoidant, and obsessive-compulsive personality disorders. Am J Psychiatry 2002;159:2036–41.

[8] Grilo CM, Shea MT, Sanislow CA, et al. Two-year stability and change in schizotypal, borderline, avoidant and obsessive-compulsive personality disorders. J Consult Clin Psychol 2004;72:767–75.

[9] McGlashan TH, Grilo CM, Sanislow CA, et al. Two-year prevalence and stability of individual DSM-IV criteria for schizotypal, borderline, avoidant, and obsessive-compulsive personality disorders: toward a hybrid model of axis II disorders. Am J Psychiatry 2005;162:883–9.

[10] Zanarini MC, Frankenburg FR, Hennen J, et al. Psychosocial functioning of borderline patients and axis II comparison subjects followed prospectively for six years. J Personal Disord 2005;19:19–29.

[11] Skodol AE, Pagano ME, Bender DS, et al. Stability of functional impairment in patients with schizotypal, borderline, avoidant, or obsessive-compulsive personality disorders over two years. Psychol Med 2005;35:443–51.

[12] Zanarini MC, Frankenburg FR, Hennen J. Mental health service utilization by borderline personality disorder patients and Axis II comparison subjects followed prospectively for 6 years. J Clin Psychiatry 2004;65:28–36.

[13] Frankenburg FR, Zanarini MC. The association between borderline personality disorder and chronic medical illnesses, poor health-related lifestyle choices, and costly forms of health care utilization. J Clin Psychiatry 2004;65:1660–5.

[14] Bender DS, Skodol AE, Pagano ME, et al. Prospective assessment of treatment use by patients with personality disorders. Psychiatr Serv 2006;57:254–7.

[15] Linehan MM. Cognitive-behavioral treatment of borderline personality disorder. New York: Guilford Press; 1993.

[16] Gunderson JG. Borderline personality disorder. Washington, DC: American Psychiatric Press; 1984.

[17] Zanarini MC, Frankenburg FR, DeLuca CJ, et al. The pain of being borderline: dysphoric states specific to borderline personality disorder. Harv Rev Psychiatry 1998;6:201–7.

[18] Zittel Conklin C, Westen D. Borderline personality disorder in clinical practice. Am J Psychiatry 2005;162:867–75.

[19] Zanarini MC, Frankenburg FR. Pathways to the development of borderline personality disorder. J Personal Disord 1997;11:93–104.

[20] Zanarini MC, Frankenburg FR, Khera GS, et al. Treatment histories of borderline inpatients. Compr Psychiatry 2001;42:144–50.

[21] Linehan MM, Armstrong HE, Suarez A, et al. Cognitive-behavioral treatment of chronically parasuicidal borderline patients. Arch Gen Psychiatry 1991;48:1060–4.

[22] Giesen-Bloo J, van Dyck R, Spinhoven P, et al. Outpatient psychotherapy for borderline personality disorder. Arch Gen Psychiatry 2006;63:649–58.

[23] Bateman A, Fonagy P. Effectiveness of partial hospitalization in the treatment of borderline personality disorder: a randomized controlled trial. Am J Psychiatry 1999;156:1563–9.

[24] Clarkin JF, Levy KN, Lenzenweger MF, et al. Evaluating three treatments for borderline personality disorder: a multiwave study. Am J Psychiatry 2007;164:922–8.

[25] Linehan MM, Comtois KA, Murray AM, et al. Two-year randomized controlled trial and follow-up of dialectical behavior therapy vs therapy by experts for suicidal behaviors and borderline personality disorder. Arch Gen Psychiatry 2006;63:757–66.

[26] Bateman A, Zanarini M. Personality disorder. In: Tyrer P, Silk K, editors. Cambridge textbook of effective treatments in psychiatry. London: Cambridge University Press; 2008. p. 659–81.

[27] Zanarini MC, Parachini EA, Frankenburg FR, et al. Sexual relationship difficulties among borderline patients and axis II comparison subjects. J Nerv Ment Dis 2003;191:479–82.

[28] Robins E, Guze SB. Establishment of diagnostic validity in psychiatric illness: its application to schizophrenia. Am J Psychiatry 1970;126:983–7.

[29] Robins LN. Deviant children grown up. Baltimore: Williams & Wilkins; 1966.

Clinical Trials of Treatment for Personality Disorders

Joel Paris, MD

Institute of Community and Family Psychiatry, Sir Mortimer B. Davis Jewish General Hospital,
Department of Psychiatry, McGill University, 4333 Cote Ste-Catherine Road,
Montreal, QC H3T 1E4, Canada

Until recently, the treatment of patients with personality disorders was largely guided by clinical experience. However, in the past decade a series of important clinical trials, both of pharmacotherapy and psychotherapy, have been conducted. Almost all of this research deals with borderline personality disorder (BPD), a diagnosis that is common in clinical settings and that presents serious and worrisome challenges [1].

Personality disorders are chronic, but often improve with time [2–4]. In fact, the prognosis for many personality disorders (PDs) is better than for most serious Axis I disorders. Since it difficult to determine whether improvement is naturalistic or the result of any specific intervention, randomized controlled trials (RCTs) are crucial.

Another observation of importance for therapy is that depressed patients who also have PDs do not respond to the same treatment methods (whether pharmacological or psychotherapeutic) as those without PDs [5]. Some have challenged this conclusion in relation to antidepressants [6], but a recent meta-analysis supported it [7]. The implication is that if clinicians avoid making Axis II diagnoses, or only diagnose PD patients with comorbid Axis I conditions, they are likely to be disappointed with the results of drug treatment. Similarly, generic forms of psychotherapy may be less effective than methods specifically developed for PDs.

PSYCHOTHERAPIES

Dialectical Behavior Therapy

Dialectical behavior therapy (DBT) is an adaptation of cognitive behavioral therapy, but is an eclectic mix of methods common to several other approaches [8]. DBT is specifically designed to target the mood instability of BPD, but also addresses impulsive behaviors. It applies behavioral analysis to incidents leading to self-injury and overdoses, teaching patients alternative ways of handling dysphoric emotions. DBT emphasizes empathic responses to distress that

E-mail address: joel.paris@mcgill.ca

0193-953X/08/$ – see front matter
doi:10.1016/j.psc.2008.03.013

provide "validation" for the inner experience of patients. The program consists of individual therapy, group psychoeducation, and telephone availability for "coaching."

DBT was the subject of one of the first randomized controlled trials of a psychotherapy designed for BPD [9]. The results, published in 1991, showed that it was clearly superior to "treatment as usual" (TAU, ie, outpatient therapy in the community). After a year, patients receiving DBT were less likely to make suicide gestures and spent less time in hospital. Although the gap narrowed at 1-year follow-up [10], patients treated with DBT continued to have a higher functional level than those who were not treated with DBT.

In the 1991 study, more than 90% of patients treated with DBT stayed in therapy for the full year. That was a remarkable finding in a patient population known for a lack of treatment compliance. The highly structured nature of DBT may be responsible. However, it should be noted that the patients in this study received free treatment, while the cohort in treatment as usual did not, and that replication studies in other centers have experienced higher rates of attrition [11–15]. But these studies also confirmed the efficacy of DBT, which is also effective in BPD patients with substance abuse [16].

The main limitation of the 1991 study was that it compared DBT to TAU, which tends to offer inconsistent follow-up. The advantage of DBT could have derived from its structure and consistency rather than from any specific form of intervention.

To address this problem, Linehan and colleagues [17], conducted a new clinical trial in which the comparison group was assigned to "treatment by community experts"–therapists in the Seattle area who identified themselves as interested in BPD, and whose fees were paid for by the research team. The results, published in 2006, found several outcomes that favored DBT: reductions in overdoses and subsequent hospitalizations within the first year of treatment. But this time there were no differences between the groups in the frequency of self-mutilation. Thus, DBT remained superior, even if its advantage was narrower.

While this research is highly encouraging, we need to determine whether its findings are generalizable to clinical settings. Selection biases affecting clinical research tend to produce samples of patients who are compliant. Since not every BPD patient will follow through with DBT, we do not know whether this treatment can be applied to all cases.

Another limitation concerns long-term efficacy. Linehan [8] had suggested that a full course of treatment could take several years, but tested only the first stage (in which parasuicidal behaviors were targeted and brought under control). We also do not know whether treated samples maintain their gains and continue to improve or whether they might relapse. Although the original cohort received therapy 15 years ago, there has been no follow up.

The largest problem for DBT is that it is resource-intensive and expensive. For this reason, more than a decade after its introduction, implementation of this treatment has been spotty. Where available, it can produce long waiting lists–not surprising for a treatment whose initial phase lasts a full year. It remains to be seen whether DBT can be dismantled and streamlined for greater clinical impact, but one recent study suggests that it can [18].

Other Forms of Cognitive Therapy

Linehan [8] developed DBT because of her experience that standard cognitive behavioral therapy was not effective for this population. Nonetheless, CBT has been subjected to clinical trials in these patients. Results using a method developed by Beck (which focuses on correcting maladaptive cognitions) have been published, but the trial was open and uncontrolled [19]. In a large RCT, Tyrer and colleagues [20], found that manualized cognitive behavioral therapy was superior to treatment as usual for the treatment of recurrent deliberate self-harm in PD patients, but was less effective for those with a diagnosis of BPD.

Recently, an RCT by Davidson and colleagues [21–23] found standard CBT to be superior to treatment as usual for BPD. The average length of treatment was only 16 sessions, but CBT had a superior outcome. A report by Weinberg and colleagues [16] of a 12-week clinical trial, found that that this brief treatment was superior to TAU in that it rapidly reduced self-harm behavior in BPD. All these findings suggest that CBT for BPD need not require several years of treatment.

Schema-focused therapy, developed by Young [24], is a hybrid of CBT and psychodynamic therapy that focuses on maladaptive schema deriving from adverse experiences in childhood. A clinical trial [25] found that improvement was equivalent to a comparison group receiving transference-focused therapy (described later in this article).

The "STEPPS" program [26] is another cognitive method providing psycho-education in a group format, designed to supplement standard therapy, and it has been subjected to a successful clinical trial.

In summary, cognitive therapy is a strong contender to be considered a standard treatment for BPD. A Cochrane review [27], applying its usual high standards of evidence, concluded that the data supporting this form of treatment are promising.

While cognitive therapy has been proposed for the treatment of other personality disorders [28], RCTs are rare and clinical guidelines unclear. For example, Emmelkamp and colleagues [29] examined the use of CBT in avoidant personality disorder, comparing it to brief dynamic therapy, yet neither method was superior to a waiting list control group.

Psychodynamic Therapies

Psychoanalysts have long been interested in treating personality disorders, but patients may not always do well with this approach. Thus, when BPD patients are offered open-ended psychodynamic therapy, most will drop out within a few months [30,31].

In the first formal study of dynamic therapy in BPD, Stevenson and Meares [32] reported improvement in 30 patients who received 2 years of a therapy based on self-psychology, and results remained stable after 5 years [33]. Since there was no control group and outcome was compared with untreated patients on a waiting list (and to the overall course of the disorder), a replication was later performed [34]; however, it was not clear how representative these patients were of clinical populations.

Mentalization-based therapy (MBT) has been tested with an RCT [35], and the good results were stable on 18-month follow-up [36]. MBT is derived from attachment theory, and based on the idea that BPD patients need to taught to "mentalize" (ie, to stand outside their feelings and accurately observe emotions in self and others). MBT makes use of a number of cognitive methods, as acknowledged by Bateman and Fonagy [37,38]. For example, mentalization resembles the concept of "decentering," long applied by CBT [28]. Since the findings of the MBT trial were obtained to a day hospital, this milieu may have accounted for some of the improvement, and MBT is currently being tested in an outpatient setting [39].

Transference-focused psychotherapy (TFP) is a somewhat different psychodynamic method that aims to correct distortions in the patient's perception of significant others and of the therapist [40]. The method has been evaluated (in a comparison to DBT) in a randomized clinical trial, with results indicating approximately equivalent efficacy [41,42].

All these findings suggest that manualized dynamic therapies can also be successful for treating BPD, provided they are well structured. The most likely reason why past therapies have often failed may be that they relied on unstructured techniques, which leave patients adrift.

The findings also suggest that different forms of psychotherapy, based on different theories, can be effective.

Group Therapy
Groups have been used either as a primary therapy, or as an adjunct to other treatments. Only one controlled trial in BPD patients comparing long-term group to individual therapy has been published, with the finding that both methods achieved similar results [43].

Psychoeducation
A recent RCT [44] described the efficacy of brief psychoeducation for a mixed group of personality disorders. Education is also an essential element of DBT [8]. It is useful to explain Axis II diagnoses to patients and to encourage them to read and browse on the Internet to obtain more information.

Whereas the families of patients have been, in the past, blamed for the development of personality disorders, therapists have come to realize they are burdened by their children's psychopathology, and can be useful allies in treatment. Gunderson [45] developed a program for psychoeducation of family members, paralleling previous work on expressed emotion in schizophrenia, but has not published data on its effectiveness.

PHARMACOTHERAPIES
Almost all the research on drugs for PDs has been on BPD.

Neuroleptics

Low-dose neuroleptics have long been used for BPD, but have many side effects. Studies of haldoperidol show that patients tend to stop taking it, probably for this reason, and that short-term effects are not maintained on 6-month follow-up [46]. Three studies of olanzapine [47–49] found reductions in impulsivity in short-term clinical trials. One study [50] found that olanzapine added to efficacy in patients also receiving DBT. However, all of these reports used small samples. Moreover, clinical improvement did not translate into remission.

Specific Serotonin Reuptake Inhibitors

It is unusual today to see a patient with BPD who is not on an antidepressant. Yet this practice is not firmly based on controlled trials.

Specific serotonin reuptake inhibitors (SSRIs) have often been used for depressive symptoms in BPD. While one study [51] reported that SSRIs reduce mood swings in BPD, most [48,52,53] suggest that SSRIs are most effective in reducing anger and impulsive symptoms. High doses (eg, 60 to 80 mg of fluoxetine) may produce reductions of self-mutilation [54], but patients can have difficulty tolerating these levels.

Research has also examined MAO inhibitors [46,55] and tricyclic antidepressants [56] in BPD, but the side effects and potential lethality of these agents on overdose have not encouraged their use.

Like neuroleptics, antidepressants "take the edge off" symptoms of BPD, but do not lead to remission of a personality disorder.

Mood Stabilizers

BPD is associated with marked affective instability, and has sometimes been thought to lie in the bipolar spectrum [57]. One reason for doubting this reformulation is that studies on mood stabilizers in BPD have produced unconvincing results. The only controlled study of lithium in BPD [58] failed to demonstrate clinical efficacy, and few clinicians would wish to use a drug that is so dangerous on overdose. Carbamazepine can reduce impulsivity [55], but is also dangerous on overdose. Controlled trials of valproate [59–61] have shown only marginal efficacy in BPD, and the data suggest that while this drug reduces impulsive aggression, it is less useful for affective instability. The best results were obtained in a small-scale trial of valproate [62], but this sample was limited to patients who were comorbid for bipolar II disorder (ie, those with clear-cut hypomanic episodes), a very atypical group that may not even justify a BPD diagnosis. Lamotrigine [63] and topiramate [64,65] have also been studied in small clinical trials in BPD patients, with some effects in reducing anger and anxiety (but not depression).

In summary, mood stabilizers are more useful for impulsivity and aggression than for mood. As we have seen, the same effect can be obtained with SSRIs and low-dose neuroleptics. Although these agents are designated as "mood stabilizers," their effects do not seem to extend very well to PDs. Efficacy is better documented in bipolar I and bipolar II; the emotional dysregulation in BPD patients may be an entirely different phenomenon [57].

Other Pharmacological Agents
Zanarini and Frankenburg [66], reported that omega-3 fatty acids were helpful for BPD symptoms (in a small sample of patients obtained by advertisement). Of course a single study is not sufficient evidence to recommend this agent for a clinical population.

Polypharmacy
A wide variety of pharmacological agents reduce impulsivity in personality disorders, but none have ever been shown to produce clinical remission. These drugs are of limited value because they were developed for other purposes, and are applied to Axis II diagnoses that probably have a different pathophysiology.

Patients receiving medication usually remain unstable—in mood, impulsive actions, and relationships. This sometimes leads to the prescription of additional agents, even if they have the same therapeutic effect (and limitations) as the original prescription. Thus, polypharmacy, a practice that is not evidence-based, is commonly applied to personality disorders, making it more likely that patients will suffer from side effects. Patients with BPD are often on four to five drugs, with at least one from each major group [67]. Unfortunately, algorithms for drug treatment in BPD, included in the American Psychiatric Association guidelines for the treatment of BPD [68], which are not based on RCT evidence, lead directly to this practice.

A recent Cochrane report [69] concluded that none of the clinical trials of drugs for BPD provides enough data to support their prescription. This being the case, it makes little sense to combine many drugs, none of which are specific to the disorder, when all of which do much the same thing.

SUMMARY
The treatment of patients with PDs is more hopeful than it was in the past. However, we have become overly dependent on pharmacological treatments, neglecting psychotherapies even when they are evidence-based. Yet there is much stronger evidence for the effectiveness of psychotherapy in PDs than for any pharmacological intervention.

The main reasons psychological therapies are not more widely used is their cost and the length of time they need to be used. But several types of therapy can be effective, and some recent evidence suggests that we may be able to provide these treatments in a briefer and more practical way [18].

Future research needs to answer other questions. First, since PDs are usually chronic, treatment research should move beyond short-term studies to examine long-term effects, and treatment effects need to be shown to be superior to naturalistic remission. Second, the effective factors common to all psychotherapies need to be more specifically identified. Third, we need to develop entirely new groups of drugs that specifically target the traits that underlie PDs.

References

[1] Lieb K, Zanarini MC, Schmahl C, et al. Borderline personality disorder. Lancet 2004;364(9432):453–61.

[2] Paris J. Personality disorders over time. Washington, DC: American Psychiatric Press; 2003.

[3] Skodol AE, Gunderson JG, Shea MT, et al. The collaborative longitudinal personality disorders study (CLPS) overview and implications. J Personal Disord 2005;19(5):487–504.

[4] Zanarini MC, Frankenburg FR, Hennen J, et al. The McLean study of adult development (MSAD): overview and implications of the first six years of prospective follow-up. J Personal Disord 2005;19:505–23.

[5] Shea MT, Pilkonis PA, Beckham E, et al. Personality disorders and treatment outcome in the NIMH treatment of depression collaborative research program. Am J Psychiatry 1990;147:711–8.

[6] Mulder RT. Depression and personality disorder. Curr Psychiatry Rep 2004;6:51–7.

[7] Newton-Howes G, Tyrer P, Johnson T. Personality disorder and the outcome of depression: meta-analysis of published studies. Br J Psychiatry 2006;188:13–20.

[8] Linehan MM. Dialectical behavioral therapy of borderline personality disorder. New York: Guilford; 1993.

[9] Linehan MM, Armstrong HE, Suarez A, et al. Cognitive behavioral treatment of chronically parasuicidal borderline patients. Arch Gen Psychiatry 1991;48:1060–4.

[10] Linehan MM, Heard HL, Armstrong HE. Naturalistic follow-up of a behavioral treatment for chronically parasuicidal borderline patients. Arch Gen Psychiatry 1993;50:971–4.

[11] Koons CR, Robins CJ, Bishop GK, et al. Efficacy of dialectical behavior therapy with borderline women veterans: a randomized controlled trial. Behav Ther 2001;32:371–90.

[12] Verheul R, van den Bosch LMC, Maarten WJ, et al. Dialectical behaviour therapy for women with borderline personality disorder: 12-month, randomised clinical trial in The Netherlands. Br J Psychiatry 2003;182:135–40.

[13] Bohus M, Haaf B, Simms T, et al. Effectiveness of inpatient dialectical behavioral therapy for borderline personality disorder: a controlled trial. Behav Res Ther 2004;42:487–99.

[14] Simpson EB, Yen S, Costello E, et al. Combined dialectical behavior therapy and fluoxetine in the treatment of borderline personality disorder. J Clin Psychiatry 2004;65:379–85.

[15] Linehan MM, Schmidt H III, Dimeff LA, et al. Dialectical behavior therapy for patients with borderline personality disorder and drug-dependence. Am J Addict 1999;8:279–92.

[16] Weinberg I, Gunderson JG, Hennen J, et al. Manual assisted cognitive treatment for deliberate self-harm in borderline personality disorder patients. J Personal Disord 2006;20(5):482–92.

[17] Linehan MM, Comtois KA, Murray AM, et al. Two-year randomized controlled trial and follow-up of dialectical behavior therapy vs therapy by experts for suicidal behaviors and borderline personality disorder. Arch Gen Psychiatry 2006;63:757–66.

[18] Stanley B, Brodsky B, Nelson JD, Dulit R. Brief dialectical behavior therapy (DBT-B) for suicidal behavior and non-suicidal self injury. Arch Suicide Res 2007;11:337–41.

[19] Brown GK, Newman CF, Charlesworth SE, et al. An open clinical trial of cognitive therapy for borderline personality disorder. J Personal Disord 2004;18:257–71.

[20] Tyrer P, Thompson S, Schmidt U, et al. Randomized controlled trial of brief cognitive behaviour therapy versus treatment as usual in recurrent deliberate self-harm: the POPMACT study. Psychol Med 2003;33:969–76.

[21] Davidson K, Norrie J, Tyrer P, et al. The effectiveness of cognitive behavior therapy for borderline personality disorder: results from the borderline personality disorder study of cognitive therapy (BOSCOT) trial [comparative study]. J Personal Disord 2006;20(5):450–65.

[22] Davidson K, Tyrer P, Gumley A, et al. A randomized controlled trial of cognitive behavior therapy for borderline personality disorder: rationale for trial, method, and description of sample. J Personal Disord 2006;200(5):431–49.

[23] Palmer S, Davidson K, Tyrer P, et al. The cost-effectiveness of cognitive behavior therapy for borderline personality disorder: results from the BOSCOT trial. J Personal Disord 2006;20(5):466–81.

[24] Young JE. Cognitive therapy for personality disorders: a schema focused approach. 3rd edition. Sarasota (FL): Professional Resource Press; 1999.

[25] Giesen-Bloo J, van Dyck R, Spinhoven P, et al. Outpatient psychotherapy for borderline personality disorder: randomized trial of schema-focused therapy vs transference-focused psychotherapy. Arch Gen Psychiatry 2006;63(6):649–58.

[26] Blum N, St. John D, Pfohl B, et al. Systems Training for Emotional Predictability and Problem Solving (STEPPS) for outpatients with borderline personality disorder: a randomized controlled trial and 1-year follow-up. Am J Psychiatry 2008;165:468–78.

[27] Binks CA, Fenton M, McCarthy L, et al. Psychological therapies for people with borderline personality disorder. Cochrane Database Syst Rev 2006;(1):CD005652.

[28] Beck AT, Freeman A. Cognitive therapy of personality disorders. 2nd edition. New York: Guilford; 2002.

[29] Emmelkamp PM, Benner A, Kuipers A, et al. Comparison of brief dynamic and cognitive-behavioural therapies in avoidant personality disorder. Br J Psychiatry 2006;189:60–4.

[30] Gunderson JG, Frank AF, Ronningstam EF, et al. Early discontinuance of borderline patients from psychotherapy. J Nerv Ment Dis 1989;177:38–42.

[31] Skodol AE, Buckley P, Charles E. Is there a characteristic pattern in the treatment history of clinic outpatients with borderline personality? J Nerv Ment Dis 1983;171:405–10.

[32] Stevenson J, Meares R. An outcome study of psychotherapy for patients with borderline personality disorder. Am J Psychiatry 1992;149:358–62.

[33] Stevenson J, Meares R, D'Angelo R. Five-year outcome of outpatient psychotherapy with borderline patients. Psychol Med 2005;35:79–87.

[34] Korner A, Gerull F, Meares R, et al. Borderline personality disorder treated with the conversational model: a replication study. Compr Psychiatry 2006;47(5):406–11.

[35] Bateman A, Fonagy P. Effectiveness of partial hospitalization in the treatment of borderline personality disorder: a randomized controlled trial. Am J Psychiatry 1999;156:1563–9.

[36] Bateman A, Fonagy P. Treatment of borderline personality disorder with psychoanalytically oriented partial hospitalization: an 18-month follow-up. Am J Psychiatry 2001;158:36–42.

[37] Bateman A, Fonagy P. Psychotherapy for borderline personality disorder: mentalization based treatment. Oxford: Oxford University Press; 2004.

[38] Bateman A, Fonagy P. Mentalization-based treatment: a practical guide. New York: John Wiley; 2006.

[39] Fonagy P. An update of on BPD treatment evaluation research in England. Presented to the NIMH international think tank for the more effective treatment of borderline personality disorder. Lincthinum (MD); December 2004.

[40] Clarkin JF, Levy KN, Lenzenweger MF, et al. The personality disorders institute/borderline personality disorder research foundation randomized control trial for borderline personality disorder: rationale, methods, and patient characteristics. J Personal Disord 2004;18: 52–72.

[41] Clarkin JF, Levy KN, Lenzenweger MF, et al. Evaluating three treatments for borderline personality disorder: a multiwave study. Am J Psychiatry 2007;164:1–8.

[42] Levy KN, Clarkin JF, Yeomans FE, et al. The mechanisms of change in the treatment of borderline personality disorder with transference-focused psychotherapy. J Clin Psychol 2006;62(4):481–501.

[43] Munroe-Blum H, Marziali E. A controlled trial of short-term group treatment for borderline personality disorder. J Personal Disord 1995;9:190–8.

[44] Huband N, McMurran M, Evans C, et al. Social problem-solving plus psychoeducation for adults with personality disorder: pragmatic randomised controlled trial. Br J Psychiatry 2007;190:307–13.

[45] Gunderson JG. Borderline personality disorder: a clinical guide. Washington, DC: American Psychiatric Press; 2001.

[46] Soloff PH, Cornelius J, George A, et al. Efficacy of phenelzine and haloperidol in borderline personality disorder. Arch Gen Psychiatry 1993;50:377–85.

[47] Zanarini MC, Frankenburg FR. Olanzapine treatment of female borderline personality disorder patients: a double-blind, placebo-controlled pilot study. J Clin Psychiatry 2001;62: 849–54.

[48] Zanarini MC, Frankenburg FR, Parachini EA. A preliminary, randomized trial of fluoxetine, olanzapine, and the olanzapine-fluoxetine combination in women with borderline personality disorder. J Clin Psychiatry 2004;65:903–7.

[49] Bogenschutz MP, Nurnberg GH. Olanzapine versus placebo in the treatment of borderline personality disorder. J Clin Psychiatry 2004;65:104–9.

[50] Soler J, Pascual JC, Campins J, et al. Double-blind, placebo-controlled study of dialectical behavior therapy plus olanzapine for borderline personality disorder. Am J Psychiatry 2005;162:1221–4.

[51] Rinne T, van den Brink W, Wouters L, et al. SSRI treatment of borderline personality disorder: a randomized, placebo-controlled clinical trial for female patients with borderline personality disorder. Am J Psychiatry 2002;159:2048–54.

[52] Salzman C, Wolfson AN, Schatzberg A, et al. Effect of fluoxetine on anger in symptomatic volunteers with borderline personality disorder. J Clin Psychopharmacol 1995;15:23–9.

[53] Coccaro EF, Kavoussi RJ. Fluoxetine and impulsive aggressive behavior in personality-disordered subjects. Arch Gen Psychiatry 1997;54:1081–8.

[54] Markowitz PJ. Pharmacotherapy of impulsivity, aggression, and related disorders. In: Hollander EE, Stein DJ, editors. Impulsivity and Aggression. New York: John Wiley; 1995. p. 263–86.

[55] Cowdry RW, Gardner DL. Pharmacotherapy of borderline personality disorder: alprazolam, carbamazepine, trifluoperazine, and tranylcypromine. Arch Gen Psychiatry 1988;45:111–9.

[56] Soloff PH, George A, Nathan S, et al. Amitriptyline versus haloperidol in borderlines: final outcomes and predictors of response. J Clin Psychopharmacol 1989;9:238–46.

[57] Paris J, Gunderson JG, Weinberg I. The interface between borderline personality disorder and bipolar spectrum disorder. Compr Psychiatry 48:145–154.

[58] Links PS, Steiner M, Boiago I, et al. Lithium therapy for borderline patients: preliminary findings. J Personal Disord 1990;4:173–81.

[59] Hollander E, Tracy KA, Swann AC, et al. Divalproex in the treatment of impulsive aggression: efficacy in cluster B personality disorders. Neuropsychopharmacology 2003;28: 1186–97.

[60] Hollander E, Swann AC, Coccaro EF, et al. Impact of trait impulsivity and state aggression on divalproex versus placebo response in borderline personality disorder. Am J Psychiatry 2005;162:621–4.

[61] Kavoussi RJ, Coccaro EF. Divalproex sodium for impulsive aggressive behavior in patients with personality disorder. J Clin Psychiatry 1998;59:676–80.

[62] Frankenburg FR, Zanarini MC. Divalproex sodium treatment of women with borderline personality disorder and bipolar II disorder: a double-blind placebo-controlled pilot study. J Clin Psychiatry 2002;63:442–6.

[63] Tritt K, Nickel C, Lahmann C, et al. Lamotrigine treatment of aggression in female borderline-patients: a randomized, double-blind, placebo-controlled study. J Psychopharmacol 2005;19:287–91.

[64] Nickel MK, Nickel C, Mitterlehner FO, et al. Topiramate treatment of aggression in female borderline personality disorder patients: a double-blind, placebo-controlled study. J Clin Psychiatry 2004;65:1515–9.

[65] Loew TH, Nickel MK, Muehlbacher M, et al. Topiramate treatment for women with borderline personality disorder: a double-blind, placebo-controlled study. J Clin Psychopharmacol 2006;26:61–6.

[66] Zanarini MC, Frankenburg FR. Omega-3 fatty acid treatment of women with borderline personality disorder: a double-blind, placebo-controlled pilot study. Am J Psychiatry 2003;160:167–9.

[67] Zanarini MC, Frankenburg FR, Khera GS, et al. Treatment histories of borderline inpatients. Compr Psychiatry 2001;42:144–50.
[68] Oldham JM, Gabbard GO, Goin MK, et al. Practice guideline for the treatment of borderline personality disorder. Am J Psychiatry 2001;158(Suppl):1–52.
[69] Binks CA, Fenton M, McCarthy L, et al. Pharmacological interventions for people with borderline personality disorder. Cochrane Database Syst Rev 2006;(1):CD005653.

Assessment and Emergency Management of Suicidality in Personality Disorders

Juveria Zaheer, MD[a], Paul S. Links, MD, FRCPC[b],*,
Eleanor Liu, PhD[c]

[a]Department of Psychiatry, University of Toronto, Mount Sinai Hospital, 600 University Avenue, Toronto, Ontario, Canada M5G 1X5
[b]Department of Psychiatry, University of Toronto, St. Michael's Hospital, 30 Bond St., Rm. 2-010d, Toronto, Ontario M5B 1W8, Canada
[c]Centre for Addiction and Mental Health, Department of Psychiatry, University of Toronto, 33 Russell St., Toronto, Ontario M5S 2S1, Canada

Previous evidence has shown a link between suicidal behavior and a diagnosis of a personality disorder, and the research is most robust regarding borderline personality disorder (BPD). This article examines the association between suicidal behavior and personality disorders in three ways. First, we update the review of epidemiological evidence for the association between suicidal behavior and suicide in individuals who have a personality disorder diagnosis, particularly in BPD. If the epidemiological evidence continues to find a strong correlation between suicide, suicidal behavior, and BPD, then the clinician is left with the challenge of differentiating patients who have BPD who are at high versus low risk of suicide. In the second part of the article, we present new empirical evidence that characterizes suicidal behavior in patients who have BPD, specifically examining patient characteristics that differentiate patients who have BPD with a history of high versus low lethality suicide attempts. Finally, based on the evidence reviewed and our clinical experience, we discuss the approach to a patient who has BPD and presents to the emergency department because of an increased risk of suicide.

EPIDEMIOLOGICAL EVIDENCE

Cluster B

Although significant epidemiological evidence exists to link personality disorders with suicidal behavior, most of this research concentrates on the Cluster B personality disorders. More limited research exists on Clusters A and C, and the evidence is reviewed according to respective clusters rather than

*Corresponding author. E-mail address: paul.links@utoronto.ca (P.S. Links).

0193-953X/08/$ – see front matter
doi:10.1016/j.psc.2008.03.007

individual personality disorders. We begin by reviewing the rates of personality disorders in subjects who have died by suicide or made suicide attempts. Then we present the rates of suicide and suicide attempts in samples of individuals with various personality disorders.

Studies have shown evidence suggesting a relationship between antisocial personality disorder (ASPD) and suicidal behavior. The DSM-IV states that individuals diagnosed with ASPD are more likely than members of the general population to die by violent means, including suicide, and ASPD has been linked with adolescent suicide behavior, including suicidal ideation, suicide attempts, and suicide. Marttunen and colleagues [1] from the Comprehensive Psychological Autopsy Study in Finland estimated that 17% of adolescents aged 13 to 19 who died by suicide met criteria for conduct disorder or ASPD. When Marttunen and colleagues [2] examined adolescents with nonfatal suicidal behavior, approximately 45% of boys and one third of girls were characterized by antisocial behavior. Beautrais and colleagues [3] studied individuals who had made medically serious suicide attempts and compared them with community comparison subjects. After controlling for the correlations between mental disorders, it was found that the risk of a serious suicide attempt was 3.7 times higher for individuals who had ASPD than for individuals who did not. When they examined men younger than age 30, the risk of a serious suicide attempt was almost nine times more likely among men with the disorder; for women, the risk of a serious attempt was 2.3 times higher.

Some studies have attempted to document the lifetime risk of suicide in a sample of individuals who have ASPD. Frances and colleagues [4] estimated the base risk of suicide completions among ASPD individuals to be 5%, with an 11% rate of attempts, which confirmed the results from Maddocks and colleagues [5], who estimated a lifetime suicide risk of 5% in a 5-year follow-up of a small sample of individuals who had ASPD.

Oldham [6] suggested that the accepted lifetime risk of 5% is low, because patients who have ASPD tend to engage in risk-taking behavior, which makes it difficult to differentiate between accidental death and suicide. Laub and Vaillant [7] examined causes of death for 1000 delinquent and nondelinquent boys followed up from ages 14 to 65 years. Deaths by violent causes (ie, accident, suicide, or homicide) were significantly more common in delinquent compared with nondelinquent boys; equal proportions of both groups, however, died by suicide.

Patients who have BPD represent 9% to 33% of all suicides [8]. Lesage and colleagues [9], in a sample of 75 men aged 18 to 35 whose deaths were declared suicides, found that 30% had BPD based on psychological autopsies. Among chronically suicidal patients with four or more visits in a year to a psychiatric emergency department, most often these patients met criteria for BPD, and they accounted for 12% of all psychiatric emergency department visits during the year studied [8]. In a study of attempters who presented to an urban hospital emergency department, 39 single attempters and 114 multiple attempters of suicide were compared regarding the diagnosis of BPD. Multiple attempters were significantly more likely to receive this diagnosis than single attempters (41.2% versus 15.4%; $P < .01$) [10]. Forman and colleagues also found that patients with multiple suicide attempts displayed more severe psychopathology, suicidality, and poorer interpersonal functioning, and these differences existed even after controlling for a diagnosis of BPD. Soderberg [11] followed 64 consecutive admissions to an inpatient unit for parasuicidal behavior (defined as all self-destructive actions with the reported intent of achieving some change in the life situation of a patient, including suicide attempts) and investigated these patients for Axis I and Axis II disorders using structured diagnostic interviews. Fifty-five percent of these patients were found to have BPD as a primary diagnosis.

BPD is the only personality disorder in the DSM-IV to have recurrent suicidal or self-injurious behavior as one of the diagnostic criteria. A history of suicidal behavior is found in 60% to 78% of patients who have BPD, with an even higher percentage engaging in self-injurious behavior. Recent research has examined risk factors for suicide and suicide behavior in patients who have BPD. In a case-control study, McGirr and colleagues [12] investigated 120 subjects who met DSM-IV criteria for BPD, 50 controls, and 70 patients who died by suicide between 2001 and 2005 and found that suicide in patients who had BPD was associated with higher levels of current and lifetime Axis I comorbidity, novelty seeking, impulsivity, hostility, and comorbid personality disorders and lower levels of harm avoidance. McGirr and colleagues [12] also determined that individuals who had BPD who suicided had fewer psychiatric hospitalizations and suicide attempts than BPD controls but were more likely to meet criteria for current and lifetime substance dependence disorders and have Cluster B comorbidity.

In a prospective trial that followed 621 patients who were assessed in semistructured interviews and followed over 2 years, Yen and colleagues [13] showed that certain diagnostic criteria of this disorder, including impulsivity, identity disturbance, and affective instability, were also significantly associated with suicidal behavior. Patients at higher risk for suicide seemed to be young, ranging from adolescence into the third decade, which likely reflects a decrease in severity of symptoms later in adulthood in most patients [8]. A recent metaanalysis by Pompili and colleagues [14] compared eight studies from 1980 to 2005 composed of 1174 patients with a diagnosis of BPD, 94 of whom died by suicide. The risk of suicide was significantly higher compared with the general population. The study also showed higher rates of suicide in short-term versus long-term follow-up, which suggested that suicide risk is highest in the initial phases of the illness rather than the chronic period [14].

The lifetime risk of suicide for patients who have BPD has been quoted to be between 3% and 10%; Paris [15] suggested that a rate of 10% has been confirmed by several cohorts, including a 15-year follow-up from the New York Psychiatric Institute and a follow-up of patients over 15 to 27 years at a Montreal general hospital but also pointed out that another major follow-up study of BPD had a much lower rate at 3%. Yoshida and colleagues [16] conducted a retrospective review of Japanese patients who received treatment in an inpatient facility from 1973 to 1989 and found that 5 of 72 patients (6.9%) had suicided, which was in keeping with the lifetime risk found in North American and European studies. Links and colleagues [17] followed 130 former inpatients with either the traits or the diagnosis of BPD and found that 6 of 130 (4.6%) died by suicide over 7 years' follow-up. In another prospective study that followed patients who had BPD over 10 years, Zanarini and colleagues [18] found a suicide rate of 4%. This lower rate may have been caused by examining a sample that agreed to follow-up and received regular treatment.

Narcissistic personality disorder is an uncommon diagnosis in community samples compared with ASPD and BPD, and the data regarding the risk of suicide in individuals who have this disorder are scarce. In samples of suicide victims studied with the psychological autopsy method, narcissistic personality disorder is infrequently identified. Apter and colleagues [19] studied 43 consecutive suicides by Israeli men aged 18 to 21; the suicides occurred during their compulsory military service. Psychological autopsies were performed using preinduction assessment information, service records, and extensive postmortem interviews. Based on this methodology, the most common Axis II personality disorders were schizoid personality in 14 of 43 men (37.2%) and narcissistic personality in 10 of 43 men (23.3%). Stone's [20] follow-up study of 550 patients admitted to the New York State Psychiatric Institute provided some information on this outcome for individuals hospitalized with narcissistic personality disorder. According to a 15-year follow-up, patients with the disorder or narcissistic traits were significantly more likely to have died by suicide compared with patients without the disorder or traits [20]. These results should be treated with caution, however, because the researcher was aware which patients had suicided when he scored them for narcissistic traits, and he did not use a standardized measure with established reliability. In more recent work, Heisel and colleagues [21] suggested that narcissistic personality has been implicated as a potential risk factor for late-life suicide. In a retrospective study, 20 patients who met criteria for narcissistic personality disorder or narcissistic traits were rated significantly higher on the Hamilton Depression Inventory suicide item than patients without, controlling for age, sex, depression, and cognitive function.

Few studies have reported on the risk of suicide or suicide attempts in individuals who have histrionic personality disorder, and studies that do comment on the relationship between this diagnosis and suicidal behavior have rarely controlled for the presence of BPD. In a psychological autopsy study of individuals aged 60 years or older, Harwood and colleagues [22] found that 4 out of 77 (5.2%) suicides in their sample had histrionic personality disorder based on ICD-10 personality disorder diagnoses, and 44% of the sample showed evidence of personality disorders or personality trait accentuation. Although the high prevalence of personality disorders in general was of interest, their method of diagnosis was not rigorous or standardized for reliability. Ferreira de Castro and colleagues [23] noted that histrionic personality disorder was the most common personality disorder diagnosis (22% of all subjects) in their sample, which was composed of individuals who engaged in self-injurious behavior but whose intent was not death.

Clusters A and C

Epidemiological evidence for the risk of suicide or suicide attempts among individuals with either Cluster A or Cluster C personality disorders is relatively scarce. Most studies do not control for coexisting BPD mediating the observed suicidal behavior of the subjects examined. Depending on the study, the prevalence of Cluster A or C personality disorders in adults who presented to an emergency department after a suicide attempt or self-injury ranges from 3% to 5% for schizoid personality disorder, 9% for schizotypal personality disorder, 8% to 10% for paranoid personality disorder, 6% to 20% for avoidant personality disorder, 1% to 9% for dependent personality disorder, and 6% for obsessive-compulsive personality disorder [8]. In their study of inpatient suicide attempters between the ages of 13 and 19, Brent and colleagues [24] reported that 27% fulfilled criteria for any Cluster A and 70% for any Cluster C personality disorder. Only a diagnosis of borderline or any personality disorder, however, was significant in this sample compared with a group of psychiatric nonsuicidal control subjects.

Analyzing data from the National Suicide Prevention project in Finland, Isometsa and colleagues [25] established personality disorder diagnoses in a random sample of 229 of the 1397 suicides studied. Isometsa and colleagues [25] determined that 1% of their entire sample of persons with a personality disorder fulfilled criteria for paranoid personality disorder, 6% for avoidant personality disorder, 7% for dependent personality disorder, 3% for obsessive-compulsive personality disorder, and 18% for Cluster C personality disorders not otherwise specified. Individuals with Cluster C personality disorders made up approximately 10% of the total random sample of 229 subjects. These patients were seemingly overrepresented considering the estimated 2% to 4% prevalence of Cluster C personality disorders in the general population [25]. Ninety-six percent of these patients experienced either comorbid depressive symptoms (74%) or substance use disorders (30%). Using a comparison group matched for age and sex, subjects with or without Cluster C personality disorders who suicided were not significantly different with respect to mood disorders, substance abuse, or previous suicide attempts [25].

Chioqueta and Stiles [26] measured the risk for suicide attempts in psychiatric outpatients with specific Cluster C personality disorders by assessing 142 patients in a psychiatric outpatient clinic for personality disorders using a structured clinical interview and correlating these findings with a history of suicide attempts. Among the Cluster C personality disorders, dependent personality disorder (35%) had the highest percentage of suicide attempts compared with avoidant (18%) and obsessive-compulsive (14%) personality disorders [26]. After logistic regression analysis to control for the presence of lifetime depressive disorder and depressive severity, these results were not statistically significant. They concluded that the assessment of suicide risk in patients with Cluster C personality disorders is less relevant than an appropriate assessment of comorbid depressive disorder history and current depression severity [26].

Studies also have reported on rates of attempted suicide and suicide among individuals diagnosed with Cluster A personality disorders. Fenton and colleagues [27] located patients from the Chestnut Lodge Follow-Up study who were originally diagnosed with schizotypal personality disorder and found that 3% had suicided, 24% had attempted suicide, and 45% had expressed suicidal ideation at some point during the previous 19 years. Among patients admitted to the psychiatric department of a German hospital between 1981 and 1994 who were assigned a primary diagnosis of personality disorder upon admission, Ahrens and Haug [28] found that 44% of individuals diagnosed with schizoid personality disorder displayed suicidal tendencies, as did 47% of the patients with paranoid personality disorder or anakastic personality disorder.

In summarizing the recent evidence, several studies have examined the link between personality disorders and suicidal behavior. Although there is some evidence for Clusters A and C and Cluster B personality disorders to be related to suicidal behavior and suicide, the strongest link still exists with the diagnosis of BPD.

CHARACTERISTICS OF SUICIDAL BEHAVIOR IN PATIENTS WHO HAVE BORDERLINE PERSONALITY DISORDER: EMPIRICAL EVIDENCE

In working with patients who have BPD, clinicians have the unwieldy challenge of differentiating patients at high risk for suicide versus patients not at high risk. In this section, we use data from a randomized controlled clinical trial of 180 participants who had BPD and recurrent suicidal behavior and present the features of suicidal behavior that typify a sample of patients who have BPD. We also partially replicate an earlier investigation by Soloff and colleagues [29] to define predictors of high-lethality suicidal behavior within a sample of patients who have BPD.

Soloff and colleagues [29] used a prospective design to assess risk factors in a sample of 113 subjects who had BPD. Their purpose was to differentiate high versus low lethality suicide attempters based on demographic, diagnostic, clinical, and psychosocial variables. Based on a median split on scores from the Medical Lethality Scale, subjects were classified as high lethality attempters for any lifetime attempt (attempts such as a sedative drug overdose defined as "comatose" or requiring hospitalization) versus low lethality attempters. The authors examined for significant predictor variables based on univariate analyses and separate regressions using variables from each content area. Then they entered the variables found to be significant into a final multivariate logistic regression model. The model was further challenged by adding back each significant variable from the content category regressions one variable at a time. The final logistic regression model found the following risk factors significantly associated with high versus low lethality status: low socioeconomic status (SES), comorbidity with ASPD, extensive treatment histories, and a high score on the Suicide Intent Scale. Soloff and colleagues [29] stressed the importance of developing predictors of high-risk suicidal behavior within a sample of patients who have BPD because this dilemma often faces clinicians in an outpatient or emergency department setting.

The purpose of the current study was to partially replicate Soloff and colleagues' [29] investigation of demographic, diagnostic, clinical, psychosocial, and treatment history characteristics that significantly differentiate high versus low lethality attempters within a sample of patients who have BPD. The participants were assessed as part of a multi-site, randomized controlled comparison of dialectical behavior therapy to a control condition, general psychiatric management, for parasuicidal adults diagnosed with BPD. Participants received continuous treatment for a period of 1 year with evaluation of outcomes every 4 months, followed by a 2-year follow-up period with evaluation every 6 months.

The primary objective of this randomized controlled trial was to assess the clinical and cost effectiveness of dialectical behavior therapy compared with that of general psychiatric management. The primary outcome measures were the frequency and severity of parasuicidal behaviors (defined as behaviors involving nonfatal self-harm that results in tissue damage, illness, or risk of death) in each of the two groups during the treatment interval and the follow-up period. Secondary clinical outcome measures included psychiatric hospitalization, psychiatric symptomatology, BPD Axis II criteria, anger expression, treatment retention, and social and global functioning.

Based on the baseline assessments of the study participants, we examined the demographic, diagnostic, clinical, psychosocial, and treatment variables that differentiated high versus low lethality attempters.

METHOD

Eligible participants met the following inclusion criteria: BPD diagnosis by International Personality Disorder Examination (IPDE) [30], at least two parasuicides within the past 5 years, at least one parasuicide in last 3 months, more than 17 years of age, and not meeting the exclusion criteria; psychotic disorder, bipolar I disorder, current active substance dependence, organic brain syndrome or mental retardation, and chronic or serious physical health problem.

Based on the rating of medical risk of death taken from the Parasuicidal History Interview (M.M. Linehan, A.W. Wagner, G. Cox, unpublished data, 1983), we divided the groups into high and low lethality categories based on maximum lifetime rating: the high lethality group scored 4 or more on the medical risk of death scale, which indicated that the risk was considered "high" (eg, "overdose of over 50 pills or 11-30 pills potentially lethal in low doses or combined with large amount of alcohol, stabbing to body; pulling trigger of a loaded gun aimed at limb etc") versus acts considered low lethality based on a score of 3 or less defined as "moderate" medical risk of death (eg, "overdose of 11-50 pills...deep cuts anywhere but neck, shoot BB gun into limb etc"). The two groups were compared on characteristics captured as part of their baseline assessments: demographics (age, sex, marital status, number of years of education, number of children), lifetime diagnoses (major depressive disorder), substance abuse, bipolar II, dysthymia, panic disorder, social phobia, special phobia, obsessive-compulsive disorder, posttraumatic stress disorder (PTSD), anorexia nervosa, bulimia nervosa, Axis II diagnoses, and the total number of Axis II disorders; clinical state and personality (Beck Depression Inventory [31], Zanarini Rating Scale for Borderline Personality Disorder) [32], number of BPD criteria, IPDE dimensional score, schizotypal dimensional score, Global Assessment of Functioning (GAF) at baseline and Social Adjustment Scale–R [33]; history of childhood abuse; and suicidal and treatment history (age of first attempt, frequency of self-harm in last 4 months, number of psychotropic medications at baseline, number of nonpsychotropic medications at baseline, number of psychiatric hospitalizations in the last 4 months, and number of medical hospitalizations in the last 4 months). Continuous variables were compared using Student's t-test (two-tailed), and categorical variables were assessed using chi-square tests. From the univariate analyses, we chose all variables that significantly differentiated the high versus low lethality attempters as independent variables for a final multiple regression analysis. For the final multiple regression analysis, we treated the rating of medical risk of death as a continuous variable (range from 1 to 6) and used this score as the dependent variable in the multiple regression analysis.

RESULTS

The 180 participants were typical of most study samples of outpatients who have BPD. They were mainly women (86% female), average age 30 years (SD = 9.7), unmarried (only 15% married or in a relationship), with at least high school education (only 12% had less than grade 12), and most were unemployed (66% were currently unemployed). Based on our definition of high versus low lethality, 89 (49.4%) participants were considered to have a lifetime history of high lethality attempts, and 91 (50.6%) were classified as having a lifetime history of low lethality attempts.

Across the whole sample, the suicidal behavior (including suicidal and self-harm acts) on average began at age 15.8 years (SD = 6.71). From the baseline assessment, only 1.67% (16/954 acts) of suicidal acts were characterized as carefully planned; the chance of intervention was usually present because only 37.7% of the acts considered the chances of intervention as remote or improbable and less than 12% of the acts were considered to have a clear expectation of a fatal outcome. According to the whole sample, only 28% of the suicide attempts in the past 4 months involved the writing of a suicide note, and 25% of the attempts in the past 4 months were accompanied by suicide threats. Somewhat surprisingly, in 61% of the suicide attempts in the past 4 months the participants endorsed hearing voices at the time of the attempt.

In Tables 1–5, we displayed the univariate comparisons of the high versus low lethality attempters. Table 1 indicates that the high lethality attempters were significantly older and had more children than the low lethality

Table 1
Characteristics of high versus low lethality attempters with borderline personality disorder: demographics

Risk factors	High lethality (n = 89)	Low lethality (n = 91)	T value/chi square, P
Age (y)	32.02 (10.69)	28.74 (8.75)	t (178) = 2.26, P = .025
Sex (females)	75 (84.3%)	80 (87.9%)	Chi square = 0.499, P = .52
Marital status (single)	57 (64.0%)	69 (75.8%)	Chi square = .97, P = .10
No. of years of education	13.44 (2.53)	13.68 (2.73)	t(178) = 0.59, P = .56
No. of children	0.68 (1.32)	0.34 (0.88)	t (178) = 2.03, P = .04

attempters. In terms of lifetime diagnoses, the high lethality attempters were significantly more likely to be diagnosed with PTSD and specific phobia and had a greater number of Axis II diagnoses. There was a trend for the high lethality attempters to be diagnosed with ASPD and anorexia nervosa more frequently than the low lethality attempters. The low lethality attempters were significantly more likely to be diagnosed with bulimia nervosa than the high lethality attempters. Although not displayed in Table 2, there were no significant differences between the groups related to bipolar II disorder, dysthymia, panic disorder, social phobia, obsessive-compulsive disorder, or other specific personality disorder diagnoses.

The high lethality attempters scored significantly higher on the total IPDE dimensional score and on the schizotypal dimensional subscale score of the IPDE than the low lethality attempters (Table 3). There were no differences between the groups in terms of depressive symptom scores or overall severity of BPD. The high lethality attempters scored significantly lower on their current GAF than the low lethality attempters, as shown in Table 3. Table 4 indicates that the high lethality attempters were characterized by more evidence of a history of childhood abuse (across all types of abuse) than the low lethality attempters.

Table 2
Characteristics of high versus low lethality attempters with borderline personality disorder: diagnoses

Lifetime diagnosis	High lethality (n = 89)	Low lethality (n = 91)	T value/chi square, P
Major depressive disorder	74 (83.1%)	70 (76.9%)	Chi square = 1.09, P = .35
Substance abuse	29 (32.6%)	27 (29.7%)	Chi square = 0.18, P = .75
PTSD	52 (58.4%)	33 (36.3%)	Chi square = 8.87, P = .004
Bulimia nervosa	6 (6.7%)	16 (17.6%)	Chi square = 4.93, P = .04
Anorexia nervosa	18 (20.2%)	9 (9.9%)	Chi square = 3.77, P = .06
Specific phobia	25 (28.1%)	14 (15.4%)	Chi square = 4.28, P = .05
Antisocial personality	8 (9.0%)	2 (2.2%)	Chi square = 3.96, P = .06
No. of axis II diagnoses	0.98 (1.12)	0.67 (0.97)	T(178) = 1.96, P = .05

Table 3
Characteristics of high versus low lethality attempters with borderline personality disorder: clinical state and personality

Measure	High lethality (n = 89)	Low lethality (n = 91)	T value/chi square, P
Beck Depression Inventory	37.10 (11.47)	35.42 (11.62)	t(165) = 0.94, P = .35
ZAN-BPD: total score	16.07 (7.02)	14.40 (5.56)	t(177) = 1.77, P = .08
No. of BPD criteria	7.11 (1.30)	7.29 (1.31)	t(178) = 0.89, P = .37
IPDE dimensional score	51.79 (21.23)	44.29 (17.56)	t(178) = 2.59, P = .01
Schizotypal dimensional score	0.79 (1.15)	0.27 (0.58)	t(178) = 3.77, P = .000
GAF baseline	49.93 (8.10)	54.81 (9.89)	t(178) = 3.47, P = .001
Social Adjustment Scale-R	2.82 (0.56)	2.79 (0.50)	t(171) = 0.32, P = .75

Abbreviations: GAF, Global Assessment of Functioning; IPDE, International Personality Disorder Examination, ZAN-BPD, Zanarini Rating Scale for Borderline Personality Disorder.

Finally, the high lethality attempters had more extensive histories of exposure to psychiatric and nonpsychiatric medication and more hospitalizations in the last 4 months (psychiatric and medical) than the low lethality attempters (Table 5). The two groups were also significantly differentiated on the maximum expectation of a fatal outcome from their suicidal behavior, with the high lethality attempters more likely to expect a fatal outcome than the low lethality group.

Table 6 summarizes the multiple regression and indicates the independent variables that explain a significant amount of the variance in the rating of medical risk of death from lifetime suicidal behavior: maximum expectation of a fatal outcome, schizotypal dimensional score, PTSD lifetime diagnosis, lower GAF at baseline, specific phobia lifetime, and the number of psychiatric admissions in the last 4 months. The independent variables were found to explain approximately 37% of the observed variance in the rating of medical risk of death from lifetime suicidal behavior.

DISCUSSION

The current findings partially replicate the findings of Soloff and colleagues [29]. In the current sample, variables related to more extensive treatment

Table 4
Characteristics of high versus low lethality attempters with borderline personality disorder: history of childhood abuse

Childhood trama questionnaire	High lethality (n = 89)	Low lethality (n = 91)	T value/chi square, P
Sexual abuse	12.93 (8.07)	10.67 (7.03)	t(175) = 2.0, P = .05
Emotional abuse	17.36 (6.61)	15.43 (5.75)	t(176)=2.08, P = .04
Physical abuse	11.85 (6.64)	9.54 (5.21)	t(176) = 2.58, P = .01
Emotional neglect	16.51 (5.44)	14.82 (5.04)	t(176) = 2.15, P = .03
Physical neglect	10.07 (4.29)	8.78 (4.02)	t(176) = 2.07, P = .04

Table 5
Characteristics of high versus low lethality attempters with borderline personality disorder: suicidal and treatment history

History	High lethality (n = 89)	Low lethality (n = 91)	T value/chi square, P
Age of first attempt	15.23 (6.90)	16.34 (6.51)	$t(176) = 1.11, P = .27$
Frequency of self-harm in last 4 mo	25.20 (46.72)	21.27 (31.09)	$t(178) = 0.67, P = .51$
No. of psychotropic medications	2.95 (1.83)	2.24 (2.03)	$t(176) = 2.46, P = .02$
No. of nonpsychotropic medications	1.74 (2.03)	1.07 (1.42)	$t(176) = 2.56, P = .01$
No. of psychiatric hospitalizations in last 4 mo	0.91 (1.34)	0.33 (0.76)	$t(178) = 3.59, P = .00$
No. of medical hospitalizations in last 4 mo	1.12 (1.57)	0.40 (0.82)	$t(178) = 3.93, P = .00$
Maximum expectation of fatal outcome	1.66 (0.59)	1.23 (0.68)	$t(178) = 2.95, P = .004$

histories (more exposure to medications and hospitalization), more evidence of psychosocial dysfunction, and evidence for greater suicide intent are convergent with Soloff and colleagues' findings. Soloff and colleagues [29] found more extensive treatment histories; lower SES and greater intent to die remained in the final model, explaining high versus low lethality status. Our results regarding differences in diagnoses between high and low lethality attempters were not consistent with Soloff and colleagues' findings. Soloff and colleagues [29] reported that ASPD was the strongest predictor of high versus low lethality attempters, which increased the risk of high lethality attempts threefold. In the current analyses, high versus low lethality attempters were more likely to demonstrate schizotypal features, be diagnosed with lifetime PTSD, and have specific phobias.

At this point, it is necessary to state the limitations of our replication of Soloff and colleagues' investigation. Our study attempted to address a similar issue differentiating within a sample of patients who have BPD at risk for high versus

Table 6
Regression model to explain variance in maximum lethality of suicide lifetime

Independent variables	b	Beta	T	P value
Maximum expectation of fatal outcome	0.379	0.260	3.456	.000
Schizotypal dimensional score	0.126	0.244	3.811	.000
PTSD lifetime	0.459	0.177	2.833	.005
GAF baseline	−0.018	−0.137	−2.155	.033
Specific phobia lifetime	0.610	0.195	3.017	.003
No. of psychiatric inpatient admissions	0.243	0.201	2.865	.005

$R^2 = 0.396$ (adjusted $R^2 = 0.374$); F change (1,160) = 8.210, $P = 0.005$

low lethality attempts. Our study differed from that of Soloff and colleagues [29] in many important ways, however. First, our definition of high versus low lethality was similar to—but not the same as—that used in the study by Soloff and colleagues, and different measures were used to assess medical risk of death. Second, although similar categories of risk factors were included, the measures used in the two studies are not equivalent. Finally, we chose to model our findings using a multiple regression analyses rather than logistic regression analyses.

Despite the methodological differences, some important inferences might be drawn from the two studies. Soloff [34] suggested that patients who have BPD who are at high risk for suicide might be suffering the "cumulative consequences of chronic illness" such as impaired psychosocial functioning, extensive treatment exposure without success, and a progression of suicidal behavior moving to more and more intent to die [35]. Our findings seem to paint a similar picture of patients at high risk for lethal suicidal behavior. The differences between the two studies regarding the risk of comorbid diagnoses are harder to resolve. Soloff and colleagues [29,34] suggested that comorbid ASPD might represent a synergy of multiple risk factors coming together in the same individuals: impulsivity and aggression, substance abuse, and the social and vocational consequences of antisocial lifestyle. Many risk factors for high lethality suicide attempts resembled those found in patients who have BPD who died by suicide [12]. Our findings regarding the influence of schizotypal features and perhaps lifetime PTSD may reflect that cognitive-perceptual symptoms, including dissociative features, might characterize patients who have BPD who are at high risk for highly lethal suicidal behavior. Previous evidence has found an association between schizotypal features and suicides in patients who have BPD, and some studies have found that patients who have BPD and have comorbidity for PTSD have more frequent histories of suicidal behavior than non comorbid patients [36,37].

In summary, patients at risk for high lethality suicidal behavior within a sample of patients who have BPD may characterize patients who are suffering a chronic illness course with significant psychosocial impairment. These patients may be demonstrating an escalating series of suicide attempts with more and more suicide intention. Clinicians remain challenged to decide which patients who have BPD require the greatest levels of care (eg, more frequent outpatient visits, involuntary hospitalizations) because of their level of risk. Further prospective research that establishes predictive variables that define the highest risk patients who have BPD are urgently needed.

MANAGEMENT OF SUICIDALITY IN THE EMERGENCY DEPARTMENT

In the first two sections of this article, we established the strong epidemiologic link between suicide, suicidal behavior, and BPD and the need for clinicians to differentiate between patients at high and low risk of suicide. Based on this evidence and our clinical experience, we turn our attention to the clinical management of suicidality in patients who have BPD who present to the emergency department. The American Psychiatric Association practice guidelines for the assessment and treatment of suicidal behavior [38] recommend conducting a complete psychiatric evaluation, assessing for suicide risk (specifically for thoughts, plans, and behaviors), establishing a multi-axial diagnosis, and estimating suicide risk. We use this framework to discuss the assessment and management of patients who have BPD who present with acute exacerbation of suicidal ideation or suicidal behavior to the emergency department.

When assessing suicidal behavior in the emergency department in a patient with chronic suicidality, it is useful to consider a model that describes "acute-on-chronic" risk [8]. This model suggests that acute stressors can increase a patient's baseline level of suicide risk. Comorbidities such as a past or current major depressive episode, substance use disorders, and history of sexual abuse can provide important information about a patient's chronic level of risk, whereas a current major depressive episode or increasing substance use can indicate acute-on-chronic risk. A thorough history of previous suicide attempts, including methods, lethality, and the context in which they occurred, aids in estimating a patient's ongoing suicide risk. A careful assessment of a plan for suicide and access to means is of utmost importance.

The epidemiological and empirical evidence outlined in the first two sections of this article are useful in assessing patients who have BPD for suicidal behavior. Clinicians should consider additional risk for suicide in patients with Cluster B comorbidity as discussed by McGirr and colleagues [12]. Comorbid ASPD, schizotypal features, lifetime PTSD, and cognitive-perceptual symptoms also may heighten suicide risk, as found in the empirical evidence presented in the second section.

The framework for suicide assessment includes the consideration of known risk factors to determine a level of risk, including age, sex, psychiatric diagnosis, and past suicide attempts. In patients who have BPD who present with an acute-on-chronic suicide risk, it is important to consider factors that are specific to the current emotional state of the patient and suggest a proximal relationship to suicidal behavior. Rudd and colleagues [39] defined a suicide warning sign as "the earliest detectable sign that indicates heightened risk for suicide in the near-term (ie, within minutes, hours or days)." Hendin and colleagues [40] described three signs that immediately precede the suicide of a patient: a precipitating event, intense affective state other than depression (eg, severe anxiety or extreme agitation), and recognizable changes in behavior patterns, including speech or actions that suggest suicide, deterioration in occupational or social functioning, and increased substance abuse.

The literature indicates that these events in patients who have BPD are often related to romantic or family relationships and legal or financial issues, and Brodsky and colleagues [41] showed that most initial suicide attempts in patients who have BPD and comorbid depression are triggered by interpersonal crises. Our research has shown that patients with high lethality attempts score significantly lower on their current GAF scale than patients with lower lethality attempts. It is important not only to assess patients who have BPD for risk factors relating to suicide but also take a history of recent events and functioning and observe for affective instability or intensity. Clinicians should observe for levels of aggression and impulsivity in patients, as discussed earlier in this article. Although many psychiatric assessment scales for suicidal ideation exist and are useful for tracking chronic levels of suicidality, their use in an acute setting to determine proximal risk of suicide is negligible.

The American Psychiatric Association [38] stresses the importance of establishing and maintaining a therapeutic alliance with patients who present with increasing suicidal ideation or behavior. Patients who have BPD, however, can present a challenge even to experienced clinicians in terms of building rapport. Bergmans and colleagues [42] discussed the emotions faced by health care providers responsible for treating patients in the emergency department who have BPD, including anxiety, anger, an absence of empathy, and frustration over repetitive behavior and a perception that patients are not appropriately using the emergency department. Patients who have BPD who present in crisis are faced with overwhelming internal stimuli; when patients are in distress, their ability to articulate how they are feeling and their problem-solving abilities are compromised. Clinicians can help de-escalate patients through the validation of emotional distress and modeling of appropriate behavior, reinforcing that seeking help was a good decision and treating the patient with respect, dignity, and empathy. When the patient has de-escalated, the clinician and the patient can begin the process of problem solving and establishing a plan of safety [42].

Patients who have BPD who present in crisis with significant anxiety or extreme agitation can be difficult to assess or de-escalate. Although studies have shown no evidence that long-term, low-dose antispychotics are more effective than placebo for reducing self-harm behaviors, these medications can be helpful in reducing a patient's anxiety and agitation in the emergency department, facilitating assessment, de-escalation of the patient, and development of a treatment plan [43].

Patients with a known diagnosis of BPD often have access to clinicians and support in the community. Patients frequently have a treatment plan with their primary caregiver that recommends going to the emergency department if the patient feels unsafe or is in crisis. In the emergency department, it is important to connect with a patient's health care team to inform them of the situation, arrange appropriate follow-up for the patient if admission is not indicated, and coordinate care with other professionals on the team.

Patients may benefit from family involvement in a crisis situation. A clinician can ask the patient which family members are helpful in times of crisis and can provide support in addressing interpersonal conflicts. Links and Hoffman [43] recommended that educating family members about restricting access to means should be incorporated into the care of all mental health patients. Hoffman and Fruzzetti [44] suggested that family psychoeducation and other interventions show early promise in the treatment for BPD.

Although it is clearly beneficial to develop a safety plan with a patient who has BPD, the evidence for contracting for safety remains mixed. It is our belief that contracting should be used only if a long-term therapeutic alliance already has been established and regular follow-up can be arranged. In the emergency department, a clinician is often meeting a patient for the first time and will not be the patient's primary caregiver in the future, which eliminates any benefit conferred by the contract.

Although patients who have BPD have a chronically higher risk of suicide than the general population, it is important to characterize their acute risk in an emergency setting and manage the risk appropriately.

SUMMARY

Several studies have illustrated a link between personality disorders, suicidal behavior, and suicide. The research is most robust in the field of BPD. BPD is a common and challenging diagnosis characterized by chronic suicidality, and we have attempted to differentiate between patients at risk for high versus low lethality suicide attempts. Although assessing and managing suicidality in patients who have BPD can be frustrating for even the most experienced clinicians, it is possible to recognize acutely elevated risk and use techniques to help create a therapeutic alliance and de-escalate the crisis situation.

Acknowledgments

The authors wish to thank Shelley McMain for her invaluable feedback on the article.

References

[1] Marttunen M, Aro H, Henriksson M, et al. Mental disorders in adolescent suicides: DSM-III-R axes I and II diagnoses in suicides among 13- to 19-year-olds in Finland. Arch Gen Psychiatry 1991;48(9):834–9.

[2] Marttunen M, Aro H, Henriksson M, et al. Antisocial behavior in adolescent suicide. Acta Psychiatr Scand 1994;89(3):167–73.

[3] Beautrais A, Joyce P, Mulder R, et al. Prevalence and comorbidity of mental disorders in persons making serious suicide attempts: a case-control study. Am J Psychiatry 1996;153(8): 1009–14.

[4] Frances R, Fyer M, Clarkin J. Personality and suicide. Ann N Y Acad Sci 1986;487: 281–93.

[5] Maddocks P. A five-year follow-up of untreated psychopaths. Br J Psychiatry 1970;116: 511–5.

[6] Oldham J. Borderline personality disorder and suicidality. Am J Psychiatry 2006;163(1): 20–6.

[7] Laub JH, Vaillant GE. Delinquency and mortality: a 50-year follow-up study of 1000 delinquent and nondelinquent boys. Am J Psychiatry 2000;157:96–102.

[8] Links PS, Kolla N. Assessing and managing suicide risk. In: Oldham J, Skodol A, Bender J, editors. Textbook of personality disorders. Washington, DC: American Psychiatric Press; 2005. p. 449–62.

[9] Lesage AD, Boyer R, Grunberg F, et al. Suicide and mental disorders: a case-control study of young men. Am J Psychiatry 1994;151(7):1063–8.

[10] Forman EM, Berk MS, Henriques GR, et al. History of multiple suicide attempts as a behavioral marker of severe psychopathology. Am J Psychiatry 2004;161(3):437–43.

[11] Soderberg S. Personality disorders in parasuicide. Nord J Psychiatry 2001;55(3):163–7.

[12] McGirr A, Paris J, Lesage A, et al. Risk factors for suicide completion in borderline personality disorder: a case-control study of cluster B comorbidity and impulsive aggression. J Clin Psychiatry 2007;68(5):721–9.

[13] Yen S, Shea MT, Stanislow CA, et al. Borderline personality disorder criteria associated with prospectively observed suicidal behavior. Am J Psychiatry 2004;161(7):1296–8.

[14] Pompili M, Girardi P, Ruberto A. Suicide in borderline personality disorder: a meta-analysis. Nord J Psychiatry 2005;59(5):319–24.

[15] Paris J. Half in love with easeful death: the meaning of chronic suicidality in borderline personality disorder. Harv Rev Psychiatry 2004;12(1):42–8.

[16] Yoshida K, Tonai E, Nagai H. Long-term follow-up study of borderline patients in Japan: a preliminary study. Compr Psychiatry 2006;47(5):426–32.

[17] Links PS, Heslegrave RJ, Mitton JE, et al. Borderline psychopathology and recurrences of clinical disorders. J Nerv Ment Dis 1995;183(9):582–6.

[18] Zanarini MC, Frankenburg FR, Hennen J, et al. Prediction of the 10-year course of borderline personality disorder. Am J Psychiatry 2006;163:827–32.

[19] Apter A, Bleich A, King RA, et al. Death without warning? A clinical postmortem study of suicide in 43 Israeli adolescent males. Arch Gen Psychiatry 1993;50:138–42.

[20] Stone M. Long-term follow-up of narcissistic personality disorder. Psychiatr Clin North Am 1989;12:621–41.

[21] Heisel MJ, Links PS, Conn D, et al. Narcissistic personality and vulnerability to late-life suicidality. Am J Geriatr Psychiatry 2007;15(9):734–41.

[22] Harwood D, Hawton K, Hope T, et al. Psychiatric disorder and personality factors associated with suicide in older people: a descriptive and case-control study. Int J Geriatr Psychiatry 2001;16(2):155–65.

[23] Ferreira de Castro E, Cunha MA, Pimenta F, et al. Parasuicide and mental disorders. Acta Psychiatr Scand 1998;97:25–31.

[24] Brent DA, Johnson B, Bartle S, et al. Personality disorder, tendency to impulsive violence and suicidal behavior in adolescents. J Am Acad Child Adolesc Psychiatry 1993;32:69–75.

[25] Isometsa E, Henriksson M, Heikkinen M, et al. Suicide among subjects with personality disorders. Am J Psychiatry 1996;153(5):667–73.

[26] Chioqueta A, Stiles T. Assessing suicide risk in cluster c personality disorders. Crisis 2004;25(3):128–33.

[27] Fenton ES, McGlashan TH, Victor BJ, et al. Symptoms, subtype and suicidality in patients with schizophrenia spectrum disorders. Am J Psychiatry 1997;154:199–204.

[28] Ahrens B, Haug HJ. Suicidality in hospitalized patients with a primary diagnosis of personality disorder. Crisis 1996;17:59–63.

[29] Soloff PH, Fabio A, Kelly TM, et al. High lethality status in patients with borderline personality disorder. J Personal Disord 2005;19:386–99.

[30] Loranger AW. International personality disorder examination (IPDE) manual. White Plains (NY): Cornell Medical Center; 1995.

[31] Beck AT, Ward CH, Mendelsohn M, et al. An inventory for measuring depression. Arch Gen Psychiatry 1961;4:561–71.

[32] Zanarini MC. Zanarini rating scale for borderline personality disorder (ZAN-BPD): a continuous measure of DSM-IV borderline psychopathology. J Personal Disord 2003;17:233–42.

[33] Weissman MM, Prusoff BA, Thompson WD, et al. Social adjustment by self-report in a community sample and in psychiatric outpatients. J Nerv Ment Dis 1978;166:317–26.

[34] Soloff PH. Risk factors for suicidal behavior in borderline personality disorder: a review and update. In: Zanarini MC, editor. Borderline personality disorder. New York: Taylor and Francis; 2005. p. 333–65.

[35] Malone KM, Haas GL, Sweeney JA, et al. Major depression and the risk of attempted suicide. J Affect Disord 1995;4:173–85.

[36] Stone MH. The course of borderline personality disorder. In: Tasman A, Hales RE, Frances A, editors. American Psychiatric Press review of psychiatry, vol. 8. Washington, DC: American Psychiatric Press; 1989. p. 103–25.

[37] Oquendo M, Brent DA, Birmaher B, et al. Posttraumatic stress disorder comorbid with major depression: factors medicating the association with suicidal behavior. Am J Psychiatry 2005;162:560–6.

[38] American Psychiatric Association. Practice guideline for the assessment and treatment of patients with suicidal behaviors. Arlington (VA): American Psychiatric Association; 2003. p. 278–97.

[39] Rudd MD, Berman AL, Joiner TE, et al. Warning signs for suicide: theory, research and clinical applications. Suicide Life Threat Behav 2006;36(3):255–62.

[40] Hendin H, Maltsberger JT, Lipschitz A, et al. Recognizing and responding to a suicide crisis. Suicide Life Threat Behav 2001;31(2):115–28.

[41] Brodsky B, Groves SA, Oquendo MA. Interpersonal precipitants and suicide attempts in borderline personality disorder. Suicide Life Threat Behav 2006;36(3):313–22.

[42] Bergmans Y, Brown A, Carruthers A. Advances in crisis management of the suicidal patient: perspectives from patients. Curr Psychiatry Rep 2007;9:74–80.

[43] Links PS, Hoffman B. Preventing suicidal behavior in a general hospital service: priorities for programming. Can J Psychiatry 2005;50(8):490–5.

[44] Hoffman PD, Fruzzetti AE. Advances in interventions for families with a relative with a personality disorder diagnosis. Curr Psychiatry Rep 2007;9(1):68–73.

Research Trends and Directions in the Study of Personality Disorder

W. John Livesley, MD, PhD

Department of Psychiatry, University of British Columbia, 2255 Wesbrook Mall, Vancouver, B.C., Canada, V6T 2A1

Since the publication of the *Diagnostic and Statistical Manual of Mental Disorders, 3rd edition* (DSM-III) in 1980, empirical research on personality disorder (PD) has increased almost exponentially [1]. There is little doubt that information about the structure, origins, and treatment of these disorders is more extensive and less speculative than when the DSM-III first appeared. Despite this progress, however, the study of PD seems to be at a crossroads and, to some extent, "spinning its wheels." The rapid accumulation of empirical data is not accompanied by a similar increase in knowledge or theoretical understanding: the many data translate into fewer facts and the results of empirical inquiry often raise more questions than they answer. It could be argued that this situation is typical of the early development of any area of enquiry and that it indicates that the field is flourishing. However, when surveying the contemporary situation it is difficult to ignore the nagging concern that many current findings and ideas will not stand the test of time. The problem is that many current data are tied to diagnostic concepts that are likely to evolve substantially in the relatively near future. These concerns are mitigated a little because most research has been on borderline, antisocial/psychopathic, and schizotypal PDs and these diagnoses probably have the greatest validity. Nevertheless, debate continues on the core features of each. Given the uncertainty about current phenotypes, it is possible that some—perhaps many—of our assumptions of recent progress are illusory and that the acquisition of more enduring data depends on establishing phenotypes that reflect the etiological structure of PD.

The problem of defining the phenotype is not specific to PD—it plagues much of psychiatry and accounts for current interest in endophenotypes—but it is especially acute with PDs. When contemplating research trends, it is useful to keep the problem of the phenotype in mind and to remind ourselves of what we hope to achieve from research efforts. Presumably the goal is

The preparation of this article was supported by Grant MOP-74635 from the Canadian Institutes of Health Research.

E-mail address: livesley@interchange.ubc.ca

0193-953X/08/$ – see front matter
doi:10.1016/j.psc.2008.03.014

a coherent body of knowledge about the structure, psychopathology, origins, and pathogenesis of PD that can form the foundation for an empirically based theory that will be useful in developing more effective treatment methods. This suggests that when considering current trends and possibly productive lines of inquiry, we need to consider both the prerequisites for the type of research needed to generate the knowledge required for theory development and the specific themes and research directions that are likely to enhance understanding of etiology, development, course, and treatment.

PREREQUISITES FOR RESEARCH

When examining the challenges of conducting the research needed for theory construction, two research questions stand out. First, what is the best way to conceptualize personality phenotypes? Second, what research designs are needed to capture the complexity of PD and generate a coherent body of knowledge?

The Phenotype Imperative

Probably the most pressing and potentially productive line of enquiry is conceptual and empirical work to define PD phenotypes and construct an evidence-based nosology. Most studies are based on global diagnoses based on DSM-IV [2] criteria sets. The limitations of DSM diagnoses are all too apparent. Most diagnostic criteria are too imprecise for satisfactory measurement. Future progress hinges on the development of a standardized nomenclature based on genetically informed constructs. Research is also handicapped by substantial overlap among DSM-IV disorders, which makes it difficult to ensure that research findings are specific to the disorder studied, and by the heterogeneity of most diagnoses—a major obstacle when investigating etiology and basic neurobehavioral mechanisms. There are also questions about the reliability and validity of many DSM-based assessment tools. Because of this combination of problems, the independent variable (the assessment and diagnosis of PD) in many studies is poorly defined, overlaps substantially with related constructs, has modest validity, and is assessed by measurement methods that show only modest agreement with each other. It is not possible to develop a solid body of knowledge in this way. The adherence to DSM categorical diagnoses is itself worthy of systematic research. It reveals how a consensus that lacks a solid scientific foundation can be maintained by sociologic processes for long periods and how it leads investigators to organize research around dubious independent variables, the kind of variable that they would reject in other circumstances.

Re-defining personality disorder phenotypes

Problems with current phenotypes suggest that an important research trend will be the use of more rigorously defined diagnostic constructs. Refinements to current diagnoses probably need to begin by developing a general definition of PD within an overarching definition of mental disorder. Definition of specific disorders would then involve specifying how the defining features of PD are expressed in each diagnosis and delineating the constellation of traits that characterize each condition [3]. This structure is similar to that of DSM-IV. The main difference is definition of the specific traits delineating each diagnosis. This would eliminate the measurement problems arising from the fact that current criteria are a confusing mixture of traits and specific behaviors. Decomposition of each disorder into its component traits would permit detailed analysis of the specific features of each disorder and help to mitigate the effects of the heterogeneity of current diagnostic constructs. It would also facilitate biological and behavioral research into underlying mechanisms because these seem to be more closely related to primary traits than to global diagnoses. The value of deconstructing diagnoses in this way is illustrated by the pharmacological treatment of borderline personality disorder (BPD): medication is usually used to target specific traits such as impulsivity, affective lability, and cognitive dysregulation rather than the global disorder [4].

A challenge in developing rigorously defined diagnostic constructs is the almost infinite variability of PD, which encourages the use of idiosyncratic constructs such as rejection sensitivity and impulsive-aggression, which makes it difficult to integrate research findings. This problem is compounded by the rich array of personality descriptors available in natural language [5]. Descriptions of PD draw upon this everyday language without developing systematic definitions of key constructs such as narcissism and impulsivity. As a result, many terms used to describe PDs are little more than folk concepts. For example, the term "impulsivity" is applied to behaviors ranging from deliberate self-harm to sensation-seeking and reckless acts that are probably etiologically and functionally distinct. At the same time, the considerable variation in overt manifestations of PD and the multidetermined nature of most behaviors makes it difficult to identify constructs that are relatively distinct and to avoid the construct drift that occurs as the meaning of constructs shifts across different uses and assessment instruments.

The trend toward the use of more rigorously defined diagnostic constructs is likely to involve the development of a systematic taxonomy of personality disorder with an attempt to anchor these constructs to underlying genetic or neurobehavioral dimensions. This would help to reduce different uses of the same term and construct drift. The research dividends arising from a systematic taxonomy of personality constructs are illustrated by the five-factor taxonomy of normal personality traits that makes the structural relationships among traits explicit. The robustness of the four-factor model of PD traits [6] suggests that this approach is likely to be useful in constructing a systematic taxonomy of PD traits that would bring order to current confusion about the meaning of many diagnostic constructs. With this approach, the primary traits of PD would be organized within a four-factor framework that would make the structural relationships among traits explicit.

Although the development of a standard nomenclature appears a daunting task, it may be more attainable than first appears. Many of the empirical findings needed for a biologically informed classification are available and the methodology needed to define diagnostic constructs is well established. First, the construction of an empirically based classification could be considered analogous to the construction of a multiple-scale personality inventory with diagnoses being equivalent to scales and diagnostic criteria equivalent to items [7]. In which case, the procedure for constructing a classification would follow the well-established principles of construct validation [8,9] that have proved so successful in personality assessment. Second, considerable progress has been made in explicating the trait structure of normal and disordered personality that could provide a useful starting point for nosological development. Third, progress is being made in linking to personality constructs to underlying biological dimensions [10] and in explicating the genetic architecture of personality [11]. Within a construct validation approach, behavioral genetic findings provide an additional source of information that could be used to establish diagnostic constructs with better convergent and discriminant validity than those in current use.

Phenotypes and endophenotypes

Problems with the current phenotypes that have made it difficult to establish replicable relationships with genetic and other biological factors has led to suggestions that greater progress would result from investigations of endophenotypes that are assumed to show a closer relationship with biological process underlying mental disorders [12]. It is generally assumed that the genetic basis of endophenotypes is easier to investigate because the effect sizes of genetic loci contributing to endophenotypes are thought to be larger than those contributing to susceptibility to disorder and the genetic architecture of endophenotypes is believed to be simpler [13]. However, a meta-analysis of genetic association studies of endophenotypes found that the genetic effect sizes of the loci are no larger than those reported for other phenotypes. A review of the genetic architecture of traits in model organisms does not support the idea that the effect sizes of loci contributing to phenotypes that are closer to the biological basis of disease are larger than those contributing to disease itself [13]. Nevertheless, studies of endophenotypes of mental state disorders are increasing and this trend it also likely to be emulated in PD research. However, it is not clear that the use of endophenotypes will yield more robust findings. Moreover, this research direction does not obviate the need to develop more refined phenotypes.

Research Methodology

The second prerequisite for generating an empirically based theory is an increase in the current trend toward more sophisticated methodologies that reflect the complexity of personality pathology and that are able to shed light on the intertwined mechanisms involved in disordered personality functioning. This involves greater use of more appropriate comparison groups, better measurement of personality variables, and more widespread use of experimental designs. Little is likely to be learned from studying single diagnoses, or personality characteristics isolation, or from the analysis of single etiological factors. Or, from studies that neglect extensive overlap with other disorders, the heterogeneous nature of the condition, and the multidimensional nature of personality pathology.

A limitation of many behavioral and biological studies is a focus on single disorders assessed in atypical clinical samples and the use of general population participants for the control condition. Hence it is often difficult to determine whether research findings are specific to the PD in question, common to other or all PDs, or a more general feature of mental disorder. Interesting information may be gleaned in the process but often it leads to misleading conclusions about the specificity of postulated mechanisms that hinders the construction of valid theoretical models. These problems are clearly illustrated by early studies on the role of childhood sexual abuse (CSA) in the development of BPD, which found higher prevalence of sexual abuse in clinical samples leading to misleading conclusions about the specificity of CSA in the pathogenesis of BPD. It was only when the prevalence of CSA in patients with BPD was compared with that of other disorders and with community samples that it became apparent that the etiological role of CSA abuse is different from original speculations [14,15].

The use of atypical samples and inadequate comparison groups is not confined to the study of CSA. Current hypotheses about the specific impairment associated with BPD include structural changes revealed by imaging studies, neurocognitive processes, impaired metacognitive functions, emotional information processing, affect regulation, and object relationships; various biological mechanisms have been proposed to account for these impairments. Although these hypotheses are interestingly plausible, many are based on studies that lacked adequate comparison groups and hence it is not possible to state with assurance that these impairments are specific to BPD.

A second aspect of methodology that is changing is assessment. Two current trends are likely to prove important. First, global diagnoses are being supplemented with more detailed dimensional assessment. This trend will probably increase given the overwhelming empirical evidence that PD phenotypes are best represented with dimensional structures. Dimensional assessment offers more differentiated assessment of diagnostic constructs that will facilitate identification of basic biological and behavioral mechanisms. Dimensional assessment also offers a way to deal with changes in diagnostic constructs that are likely to occur with the compilation of evidence-based classifications. Major changes in the classification of PD create the problem of how existing knowledge about PD that is largely based on current diagnoses could be accommodated within a new system. The assessment of a comprehensive set of dimensions in addition to traditional diagnoses would permit reanalysis of existing data sets using combinations of dimensions that match any new diagnostic entities that may be proposed as a result of the classification of PD evolving into a more valid system. Second, given the uncertainty surrounding the validity of current diagnostic constructs, modest agreement across measures, and the high correlations among measures of different disorders, it seems prudent to use multiple measures of each diagnostic construct and related constructs. Such a multitrait–multimeasure approach to assessment should prove useful in refining diagnostic constructs and in identifying factors that are specific to a given diagnostic construct.

A final research trend that should be noted is the modest increase in experimental studies that have occurred in recent years. Research on PD has been dominated by descriptive studies that largely report on the covariation between diagnostic constructs and their relationship with a range of other variables. Although these studies have greatly enriched our understanding, they are less informative about underlying mechanisms.

ETIOLOGY AND DEVELOPMENT

Ideas about the causes of PD have changed substantially recently. Once thought to be primarily a psychosocial disorder, it is now recognized that a wide range of biological, psychosocial, and cultural factors contribute to its development. Most of these factors appear to have a relatively small effect and none appear necessary or sufficient to cause the disorder. Despite this progress, etiological research is only beginning to recognize that PD arises from the interplay among etiological factors and that the PDs are best explained by the stress-predisposition model [16] in which the effects of stressors are influenced by underlying genetic factors that appear to be continuous with those underlying normal personality variation.

Genetic and Environmental Influences

Until recently, discussions of the origins of PD tended to focus on the relative importance of genetic and environmental influences and emphasize the contribution of psychosocial adversity. The nature versus nurture debate assumes that genetic and environmental influences make separate and independent contributions to pathological outcomes. However, behavioral genetics studies that parse individual differences in disorders and traits into genetic and environmental influences have radically changed our understanding of the interrelationships between nature and nurture [17]. The results of these inquiries form a consistent pattern. All quantitatively variable personality and PD traits are subject to substantial genetic influence with heritability estimates typically in the 40% to 60% range. Environmental influences are largely confined to non-shared effects; that is, influences that are specific to a given member of a twin pair, eg, differential peer relationships. The exception to this pattern is criminality, which shows substantial common environmental effects; that is, influences common to both members of a twin pair such as the same family environment.

These findings are influencing research in several ways. First, they challenge assumptions implicit in many clinical theories of PD that genetic and environmental factors operate as independent main effects. The genetic predispositions that give rise to primary traits lead to the establishment of cognitive structures and processes that influence what aspects of the environment are noticed and given attention [18]. For example, inherited mechanisms underlying the attachment system selectively highlight environmental events that are relevant to attachment. In this sense, genetic predispositions help to create the environments to which they respond. Environmental influences then modify these heritable structures. Consequently, genetic and environment influences are inextricably intertwined. Thus, progress in explicating the etiology of PD is more likely to result from investigations of the interplay among genetic and environmental variables and the way psychosocial stressors are modulated by heritable characteristics than from studies of single etiological factors or combinations of related factors.

Second, behavioral genetic findings challenge the common assumption that personality is influenced by differences between families. Heritability analyses show that such common environmental effects are not significant except for antisocial behavior. Identification of nonshared influences on PD promises to be an important but challenging area of research. To date, studies of nonshared effects have been disappointing and relatively little is known about the nature of these influences. Most of these studies have been based on nonclinical samples, and clinical theories have had little influence on the selection of nonshared factors to investigate. However, the clinical literature is replete with ideas about the kind of environmental factors thought to contribute to PD that could inform studies of nonshared influences.

Third, an emerging line of research that promises to contribute to the foundations for a theory of PD is the study of the mechanisms involved in the interplay between genetic and environmental influences: gene-environment interaction and gene-environment correlation.

Gene-Environment Interplay

Gene-environment correlation refers to genetic influences on exposure to environments. As noted previously, behavioral genetics research suggests that people create the environments to which they react to a far greater extent than originally thought because genetic factors influence both perception of the environment and the individual's choice of situations and relationships. As a result, genetic predispositions are correlated with environmental factors. This correlation may be passive, evocative, and active [19]. Passive effects occur when heritable parental characteristics give rise to behaviors that influence the child's environment so that it correlates with the child's genetic tendencies. For example, a parent with a predisposition toward that emotional lability associated with BPD may create an unstable environment that correlates with the same trait in the child, thereby increasing the risk of developing the disorder. Evocative or reactive effects occur when heritable characteristics lead to actions that evoke reactions from others that correlate with these characteristics. For example, a paranoid individual may act in a distrustful manner that elicits similar responses from others, which are then interpreted as confirmation that his or her suspicions are justified. Active gene-environment correlation occurs when individuals select or interpret environments on the basis of genetic influences, as when a person with a genetic predisposition to sensation seeking seeks out stimulating environments. Essentially, individuals select or create personal niches that correlate with their genetic tendencies. Although the contribution of gene-environment correlation to PD has not been extensively investigated, these effects are likely to be substantial: the evidence suggests that personality affects the risk of developing psychopathology by influencing perception of, and exposure to, life events [20]. These mechanisms are likely to play an important role in maintaining the repetitive patterns of maladaptive behavior that are the hallmarks of PD.

Gene-environment interaction refers to genetic sensitivity to environments—the same genetic factor may be expressed differently in different environments. Originally, gene-environment interaction was assumed to be relatively unimportant [17]. However, recently it has became apparent that genetic factors play a major role in how the individual responds to environmental conditions, and this is likely to prove a productive avenue of research. Gene-environment interaction underlies the stress-predisposition model of PD, which assumes that genetic predispositions modulate influence reaction to environmental adversity [16]. An example of gene-environment interaction is provided by Caspi and colleagues' [21] study of antisocial behavior. Childhood maltreatment, specifically erratic, coercive, and punitive parenting, is a major risk factor for the development of conduct disorder, antisocial behavior, and violent offending in boys. However, not all maltreated children develop antisocial behavior. Caspi and colleagues noted that the monoamine oxidase A gene (MAOA) is associated with aggressive behavior. This led to the hypothesis that the MAOA genotype modulates the effects of maltreatment. In a study on a large sample of children from Dunedin, they found that maltreated children with the genotype that conferred high levels of MAOA expression were less likely to develop antisocial behavior.

Developmental Pathways

The mechanisms of gene-environment interaction and correlation provide a context for conceptualizing and organizing developmental studies. Although developmental psychopathology is an active area of research, studies of the development of PD are at an early stage. The multidimensional etiology of PD suggests that varied pathways lead to the emergence of disorder with substantial individual variation in risk factors. An understanding of these pathways would be useful in developing more effective treatment methods. Currently a major gap in explanations of the emergence of PD is an understanding of the mental mechanisms through which adversity exerts a lasting influence of personality functioning. Several models have been proposed, but most are speculative and empirical research is sparse. Presumably, adversity operates in the context of heritable dispositions through the mechanisms of gene-environment interplay to modulate trait expression and influence the actual behaviors through which genetic predispositions are expressed. Early adversity also seems to lead to impaired emotion regulation and the formation of cognitive structures and processes that influence the way events, especially interpersonal events, are interpreted. Some of the cognitive therapies describe the maladaptive schemata associated with the different forms of PD but more systematic empirical studies are needed along with the studies of the environmental factors that contribute to the development of maladaptive cognitive contents and processes. There is a need for longitudinal studies of the interaction between adversity and personality traits to establish the developmental pathways that lead to disorder and the interplay between genetic predispositions and environmental factors to elucidate the contribution of gene-environment interaction and correlation in the development of PD.

Neurobiology

A rapidly expanding area of research focuses on the biological substrates of PD. This work has begun to reveal structural and functional impairments associated with a range of disorders, especially schizotypal, borderline, and psychopathic PDs. This work is likely to lead to an improved understanding of basic mechanisms and hence better treatments. Earlier studies provided evidence of the neurobiological and genetic correlates of PDs and their constituent traits. Much of this work was largely descriptive and more phenomenological in nature. It also tended to yield correlations between biological and personality variables that were modest–typically in the 0.3 range. Nevertheless, this early work counterbalanced the heavy emphasis placed on psychodynamic mechanisms in understanding the origins and functioning of PD and hence encouraged a more eclectic approach to etiology and treatment. More recently, however, research has moved beyond studies of neurobiological correlates of personality traits to explicate the brain structures and mechanisms involved in important personality processes.

Evidence of a substantial heritable component to all aspects of PD based on behavioral genetics studies initially seemed to imply that molecular genetics would make a substantial advance in understanding the origins of PD and the mechanisms involved by identifying specific genes. Although some progress has been made in identifying specific genes associated with some personality traits, progress has not been as rapid as initially expected. Results have been difficult to replicate and the genes studied explain only small amounts of observed variance. Probably more productive lines of inquiry, at least in the short term, are neuorochemical research directed toward explicating the neurotramsitter systems implicated in major dimensions of PD and neurophysiological, neuroimaging, and neurocognitive studies of neural mechanisms.

Several lines of investigation appear to be promising. First, studies of the specific brain mechanisms involved in the regulation and control of personality systems that are central to understanding PD, especially the neurocognitive mechanisms involved in emotion regulation and impulse control, the way these mechanisms are impaired in PD, and the factors contributing to these impairments. Second, investigation of the neurotransmitter systems associated with specific traits. Promising progress is being made in neurochemical and neuropharmacological research on neurotransmitters involved in emotion regulation, impulse control, and cognitive dysregulation. This area of research is likely to benefit from improved definition of phenotypes and deconstruction of major disorders into basic dimensions. Third, especially interesting are studies of how environmental factors influence neurotransmitter systems to affect the expression of specific traits. The extensive impact of environmental adversity on personality is well established but until recently it was not clear how adversity had a lasting impact. However, psychobiological studies including structural and functional imaging, neurocognitive studies, and pharmacological research are showing that early adversity appears to exert a lasting influence on the neural mechanisms involved in emotion regulation and stress responsivity and how these factors, in turn, influence information processing and other cognitive mechanisms.

LONGITUDINAL COURSE

Over the past decade, longitudinal studies have contributed new insights into the course of PD by reporting considerable temporal instability in PD diagnoses [22–24]. For example, the Collaborative Longitudinal Study [25] found that more than half of the patients assessed showed less than two criteria of their baseline disorder for at least 12 consecutive months [25]. More stability was observed when PD diagnoses were represented as dimensions. Individual diagnostic criteria also differed substantially in temporal stability. These levels of change have prompted the suggestion that PD should be considered an acute rather than a chronic disorder [26].

This conclusion contrasts sharply with previous assumptions about the stability and chronicity of PDs. PD appears to share several characteristics with classical chronic disorders: they are etiologically complex, fluctuate in severity with periods of acute distress interspersed with periods of relative stability, and outcome varies substantially across cases [27]. The findings of longitudinal studies appear to question these assumptions. However, the Collaborative Longitudinal Study [25] also found that personality traits were more stable than diagnoses and that maladjustment was also stable, although the prevalence of DSM diagnoses decreased over time. These are important but puzzling findings. They suggest that DSM diagnostic criteria sets are poor indicators of pathology as indexed by maladjustment. Consequently, it is unclear whether the significant change observed by the longitudinal studies reflects clinically important changes or merely problems with DSM criteria sets and the conceptualization of PD. These findings point to the need for further conceptual analysis of the concept of PD and the need for a new generation of longitudinal studies less closely tied to DSM-IV criteria sets to study change and stability across the various domains of personality pathology.

TREATMENT: MOVING BEYOND THE RACE TRACK

Over the past 2 decades, treatment has improved with development of manualized treatments and empirical evaluation of some common therapies. Much of this work has focused on the treatment of BPD and, to a lesser extent, psychopathy. With BPD, evidence from randomly controlled trials suggests that dialectical behavior therapy, schema-focused therapy, transference-focused therapy, mentalizing-based therapy, and medication produce significant change. The different forms of psychotherapy tend to be considered alternative ways to treat BPD. This has led comparative trials that pit different treatments against each other. There are, however, good reasons to question whether such "horse races" are the most effective ways to improve treatment. Outcome studies suggest that change primarily involves the symptomatic component of the disorder and quality of life, and that outcome does not differ substantially across therapies. This situation is similar to that reported for psychotherapy generally: meta-analyses show similar outcomes across different therapies [28,29]. The different therapies appear to incorporate common change mechanisms involving a relational and supportive component based on the therapeutic relationship and a technical component that promotes new learning and provides opportunities to apply new skills [30,31]. There is no reason to assume that the treatment of PD differs from this pattern.

Research also suggests that outcome is domain specific, with some treatment methods being more effective with some domains of psychopathology than others. With BPD, the different therapies advance remarkably different explanations of the primary impairment involved. Postulated impairments include maladaptive schema, object relationships, emotional dysregulation, and metacognitive processes, and BPD is variously considered an emotional, behavioral, cognitive, and interpersonal disorder. This means that therapies differ substantially in their primary targets for change and hence in the treatment methods used; however, all these impairments are associated with BPD. This means that current treatments are not comprehensive in the sense that they address all aspects of borderline pathology. However, since most treatments appear to incorporate effective treatment methods, the tendency to treat patients with one form of therapy means that effective methods are often not used simply because they "belong" to a different therapeutic model. For example, the methods used in cognitive therapy and dialectical behavior to improve emotional reactivity by building emotional regulation skills and emotional tolerance are not used by other treatments even though they appear effective. Considering the limited efficacy of contemporary treatments, this stovepipe approach seems counterproductive.

If different treatments produce similar but limited amounts of change and all effective therapies incorporate effective methods, little is likely to be learned from further studies comparing different therapies. Rather than selecting among treatments with comparable outcomes, it may be more productive to adopt an integrated approach that decomposes disorders such as BPD into their constituent domains of psychopathology and then selects treatment methods to address these domains from the various forms of therapy based on evidence of what works [32,33].

These ideas suggest two lines of inquiry that are likely to lead to improved treatment. First, given the major contribution that generic change mechanisms common to all effective treatments make to outcome variance, it is important to identify the optimal ways to operationalize generic mechanisms when treating PD and explicate the mechanisms through which they bring about change. Second, evidence that outcome is domain specific suggests that it is important to identify the most effective treatment methods for each domain. The features of PD include symptoms, situational problems and life circumstances, dysregulated emotions and impulses, maladaptive traits, maladaptive interpersonal behaviors, and self-pathology. It is highly improbable that the same treatment strategies will be effective for all domains.

Besides these research themes, current treatments do not adequately address two major challenges in treating PD: patient retention and motivation. Research and clinical experience suggests that many patients, perhaps as many as 50%, drop out of therapy in the first 6 months. For example, in a comparative trial of transference-focused therapy versus schema-focused therapy for BPD, 38.6% of participants were lost to therapy and assessment [34]. In addition, many patients eligible for treatment do not accept treatment. In the above study, 85 of the 173 patients screened for eligibility were excluded for various reasons. These included 40 patients who declined to participate and 2 who could not make themselves available for treatment although they met study criteria. Hence, 58.5% of eligible patients either declined or dropped out of treatment. This problem is mirrored in most outpatient and community health services creating an urgent need for innovative research on the factors associated with drop out and motivation for change.

Although few studies have explicitly addressed this problem, the literature contains hints that may be worth pursuing. It appears from the Giessen-Bloo and colleagues [34] and other studies that there are fewer dropouts in the early months of treatment with cognitive therapy than with psychoanalytically based treatments. This raises the question of what it is about the cognitive therapies that makes them more successful in retaining patients. One possible factor is the emphasis cognitive therapies place on working with patients to establish specific and attainable treatment goals. This probably helps to build the therapeutic relationship, enhance patient motivation, and promote early changes. Cognitive-behavioral therapies also seem to place greater emphasis on explicit methods to provide support and validation, which help to build the therapeutic relationship. This emphasis contrasts with the more interpretative style of some psychoanalytic therapies that places greater strain on the relationship especially early in treatment.

FORESTS AND TREES: THE IMPORTANCE OF THE "BIG PICTURE"

With increased use of sophisticated methodologies and experimental analyses that are shedding light on neurobehavioral structures and processes, it is easy to conclude that this kind of "reductionism" will be sufficient to explain personality pathology. There is little doubt that an understanding of these structures and processes as revealed by functional imaging, neurobiological studies, and neurocognitive investigations will help to delineate underlying mechanisms and bring greater coherence to our understanding of PD. However, although these developments are necessary to explain personality pathology, they are unlikely to be sufficient.

Most theories of personality emphasize both the structures and processes that comprise the personality system and the organized and coherent nature of personality functioning. The integrative mechanisms contributing to organization and coherence appear to be severely disrupted in PDs. Important aspects of personality are also concerned with meaning–the meaning individuals impose upon interpersonal events and the knowledge structures used to organize an understanding of self and the world. A full account of PD requires not only a detailed description of the specific neurobehavioral structures and mechanisms involved in disordered personality functioning, but also an account of the more molar processes involved in the integration and synthesis of higher-order processes and structures. An account of these integrative mechanisms and meaning systems is likely to require analyses and constructs at a different level of description and explanation than those concerned with explicating basic processes and specific mechanisms. Consequently, it is important not to lose sight of the importance of studying these integrative aspects of personality and the way they are impaired in PD.

At the heart of PD are fundamental problems in how individuals understand and conceptualize the self. Most theories of PD, especially theories of BPD, describe a poorly developed, fragmented, and unstable self-system. Theories also suggest that the self-system contributes to the integration of personality and to the consistency and coherence of normal functioning; however, there are few empirical analyses of self-pathology in PD. Descriptive studies of the nature of self-pathology are limited and there are even fewer studies of the integrative mechanisms that contribute to the development of the self, the pathways along which it develops, or the factors that lead to impaired structure and functioning. This information is crucial for constructing a coherent theory of PD and effective treatment methods to help patients build a more adaptive understanding of themselves and others.

References

[1] Blashfield RK, Intoccia V. Growth of the literature on the topic of personality disorders. Am J Psychiatry 2000;157(3):472–3.

[2] American Psychiatric Association. Diagnostic and statistical manual of mental disorders (DSM-IV). 4th edition. Washington, DC: American Psychiatric Association; 1994.

[3] Livesley WJ. A framework for integrating dimensional and categorical classifications of personality disorder. J Personal Disord 2007;21:199–224.

[4] Soloff PH. Psychopharmacology of borderline personality disorder. Psychiatr Clin North Am 2000;23:169–90.

[5] Allport GW, Odbert HS. Trait-names: a psycho-lexical study. Psychol Monogr 1936; No. 211.

[6] Widiger T, Simonsen E. Alternative dimensional models of personality disorder: finding a common ground. J Personal Disord 2005;19:110–30.

[7] Blashfield RK, Livesley WJ. A metaphorical analysis of psychiatric classification as a psychological test. J Abnorm Psychol 1991;100:262–70.

[8] Livesley WJ, Jackson DN. Guidelines for developing, evaluating, and revising the classification of personality disorders. J Nerv Ment Dis 1992;180:609–18.

[9] Loevinger J. Objective tests as instruments of psychological theory. Psychol Rep 1957;3:635–94.

[10] Depue RA, Lenzenweger MF. A neurobehavioral dimensional model. In: Livesley WJ, editor. Handbook of personality disorders. New York: Guilford Publications; 2001. p. 136–76.

[11] Livesley WJ. Behavioral and molecular genetic contributions to a dimensional classification of personality disorder. J Personal Disord 2005;19:131–55.

[12] Siever LJ, Torgersen S, Gunderson JG, et al. The borderline diagnosis III: identifying endophenotypes for genetic studies. Biol Psychiatry 2002;51(12):964–8.

[13] Flint J, Munafò MR. The endophenotype concept in psychiatric genetics. Psychol Med 2006;37:163–80.

[14] Fossati A, Madeddu F, Maffei C. Borderline personality diosorder and childhood sexual abuse: a meta-analytic study. J Personal Disord 1999;13(3):268–80.

[15] Paris J. Psychosocial adversity. In: Livesley WJ, editor. Handbook of personality disorders. New York: Guilford Publications; 2001. p. 231–41.

[16] Paris J. Nature and nurture in psychiatry: a predisposition-stress model of mental disorders. Washington, DC: American Psychiatric Press; 1999.

[17] Rutter M. Gene-environment interdependence. Dev Sci 2007;10(1):12–8.

[18] Livesley WJ, Jang KL. The behavioral genetics of personality disorder. Annu Rev Clin Psychol 2008;4:1–28.

[19] Plomin R, DeFries JC, Loehlin JC. Genotype-environment interaction and correlation in the analysis of human behavior. Psychol Bull 1977;84(2):309–22.

[20] Saudino KJ, Pedersen NL, Lichtenstein P, et al. Can personality explain genetic influences on life events? J Pers Soc Psychol 1997;72:196–206.

[21] Caspi A, McClay J, Moffitt T. Role of genotype in the cycle of violence in maltreated children. Science 2002;297(5582):851–4.

[22] Cohen P, Crawford TN, Johnson JG, et al. The children in the community study of developmental course of personality disorder. J Personal Disord 2005;19(5):466–86.

[23] Lenzenweger MF. The longitudinal study of personality disorders: history, design considerations, and initial findings. J Personal Disord 2006;20:645–70.

[24] Lenzenweger MF, Johnson MD, Willett JB. Individual growth analysis illuminates the stability and change in personality disorder features: the longitudinal study of personality disorders. Arch Gen Psychiatry 2004;61:1015–24.

[25] Skodol AE, Gunderson JG, Shea MT, et al. The collaborative longitudinal personality disorders study (CLPS): overview and implications. J Personal Disord 2005;19(5):487–504.

[26] Zanarini MC, Frankenburg FR, Hennen J, et al. The McLean study of adult development (MSAD): overview and implications of the first six years of prospective follow-up. J Personal Disord 2005;19:505–23.

[27] Paris J. Personality disorders over time: precursors, course and outcome. J Personal Disord 2003;17(6):479–88.

[28] Beutler LE. Have all won and must all have prizes? Revisiting Luborsky, et al's verdict. J Consult Clin Psychol 1991;59:226–32.

[29] Luborsky L, Singer B, Luborsky L. Comparative studies of psychotherapies. Arch Gen Psychiatry 1975;32:995–1008.

[30] Lambert MJ. Psychotherapy outcome research: implications for integrative and electical therapists. In: Norcross JC, Goldfried MR, editors. Handbook of psychotherapy integration. New York: Basic Books, Inc; 1992. p. 94–129.

[31] Lambert MJ, Bergen AE. The effectiveness of psychotherapy. In: Bergin AE, Garfield SL, editors. Handbook of psychotherapy and behavior change. 4th edition. New York: John Wiley & Sons, Inc; 1994. p. 143–89.

[32] Livesley WJ. Practical management of personality disorder. New York: Guilford Publications; 2003.
[33] Livesley WJ. An integrated approach to the treatment of personality disorder. Journal of Mental Health 2007;16:131–48.
[34] Giessen-Bloo J, van Dyck R, Spinhoven P, et al. Outpatient psychotherapy for borderline personality disorder: randomized controlled trial of schema-focused therapy vs transference-focused psychotherapy. Arch Gen Psychiatry 2006;63(6):649–58.

INDEX

A

Adolescence, assessment in, 482–483
  comorbidity of Axis I disorders in, 486–488
  personality disorder in, prognostic implications of, 488–489

Amygdala, in borderline personality disorder, 447, 451
  in psychopathy, functional impairment of, 466–467

Anterior cingulate gyrus, in borderline personality disorder, 443–444, 447, 449–450
  in psychopathy, 468

Antidepressants, for borderline personality disorder, 509

Antipsychotics, for borderline personality disorder, 509

Antisocial personality disorder (APD), adolescent suicidality in, 528
  assessment of, in childhood, 480–481
  change in, 513
  genetic epidemiologic study methods for, 425

Assessment, in adolescence, 482–483
  in childhood, of antisocial personality disorder, 480–481
    of borderline personality disorder, 481–482
  in children, 482–483
  methodologic considerations in, 405–409
    Axis I disorders in, 406
    diagnostic evaluation, 406–408
    impact on prevalence, 408, 416–417
    inclusion, 409
    instruments, 408
    interview in, 408–409
    psychiatric state, 406
    source of information, 416
    timing, 406
  of suicidality, **527–543**

Attachment, early problems in, as risk factor, 484

Axis I disorders, impact on, Children in the Community study, 497–498
    Collaborative Longitudinal Personality Disorders Study, 501
  predictive and comorbid, in adolescents, 486–488

B

Behavior, impact on, Children in the Community study, 497
    Collaborative Longitudinal Personality Disorders Study, 500

Biological study, of borderline personality disorder, 442–452
  of schizotypal personality disorder, 452–453
  recent advances in, **441–461**

Borderline personality disorder (BPD), assessment of, in childhood, 481–482
  biological research in, 442
    amygdala in, 447, 451
    anterior cingulate gyrus in, 444–445, 450
    hippocampus in, 448, 451
    neuroimaging in, 444–445
    opiate neurocircuitry findings in, 444
    orbital frontal cortex in, 444–445
    serotonergic system findings in, 442–444
  change in, **505–515**
    acceptance of past in, 512–514
    future orientation for, 512–513
    psychosocial, 506
    symptomatic, 505–506
  core problem in, 507–508
  group therapy for, 520
  inner pain in, 507
    lessening of, 510–511
    validation of, 510
  interpersonal strategies in, 507–508
  key features of, 507
  learning to be straightforward, clarification in, 511
    relationships in, 511–512
    vocational responsibilities in, 511

Note: Page numbers of article titles are in **boldface** type.

0193-953X/08/$ – see front matter
doi:10.1016/S0193-953X(08)00063-4